Machine Learning and IoT Applications for Health Informatics

Editors

Pijush Samui
Professor, Department of Civil Engineering
Patna, Bihar, India

Sanjiban Sekhar Roy
Professor, School of Computer Science and Engineering
Vellore Institute of Technology, Tamil Nadu, India

Wengang Zhang
Professor, School of Civil Engineering
Chongqing University, Chongqing, China

Y H Taguchi
Professor, Department of Physics
Chuo University, Tokyo, Japan

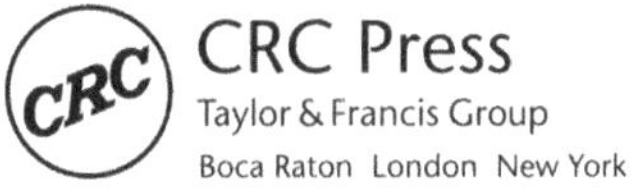

CRC Press is an imprint of the
Taylor & Francis Group, an **informa** business

First edition published 2025
by CRC Press
2385 NW Executive Center Drive, Suite 320, Boca Raton FL 33431

and by CRC Press
4 Park Square, Milton Park, Abingdon, Oxon, OX14 4RN

CRC Press is an imprint of Taylor & Francis Group, LLC

Library of Congress Cataloging-in-Publication Data (applied for)

ISBN: 978-1-032-54450-2 (hbk)
ISBN: 978-1-032-54457-1 (pbk)
ISBN: 978-1-003-42498-7 (ebk)

DOI: 10.1201/9781003424987

Typeset in Times New Roman
by Prime Publishing Services

This book is dedicated to my wife
Archita Roy

—Sanjiban Sekhar Roy

This book is dedicated to my wife
Rituparna Samui

—Pijush Samui

Preface

This book brings together leading experts from around the world to explore the transformative potential of Machine Learning (ML) and the Internet of Things (IoT) in healthcare. It provides a platform for studying a future where healthcare becomes more precise, personalized, and accessible for all. The book covers recent advancements that will shape the future of healthcare. Discover how artificial intelligence is revolutionizing disease detection, from analyzing chest X-rays for pneumonia to solving the secrets of our genes. The book investigates the transformative potential of smart devices, real-time analysis of heart data, and personalized treatment plan creation.

The book shows how ML and IoT work and presents real-world examples of how they're leading to earlier diagnoses and personalized treatments. Whether you're a researcher, healthcare professional, data scientist, or simply someone passionate about the future of healthcare, this book is an invaluable resource. Start reading and discover the exciting possibilities that lie ahead at the crossroads of ML, IoT, and health informatics.

Keep reading, learning, and inquiring.

May 2024

Pijush Samui
Sanjiban Sekhar Roy
Wengang Zhang
Y H Taguchi

Contents

Preface v

1. Machine Learning and the Role of IoT in Health Informatics 1
Burak TAŞCI
2. Bioconductor Packages to Perform Tensor Decomposition Based Unsupervised Feature Extraction 18
Y-h. Taguchi
3. Smart Health: Advancements in Machine Learning and the Internet of Things Solutions 31
Narasimha Rao Vajjhala and Philip Eappen
4. A Study Aimed at Presenting Methodologies for Enhancing Cost Efficiency in Healthcare Systems Based on Internet of Things (IoT) by Incorporating Sophisticated Deep Learning and Artificial Intelligence Techniques 52
Oishik Ghosh
5. Transforming Healthcare through Machine Learning and the Internet of Things 76
Faridoddin Shariaty
6. IoT-powered AI for Precise Pneumonia Detection in Chest X-Rays 110
Sanjiban Sekhar Roy, Mohd Anas, Abhishek Kumar Pandey, Ramanathan L. and Kathiravan Srinivasan
7. Tensor Decomposition in Genomics 131
Y-h. Taguchi
8. IoT, Artificial Intelligence and Cyber Security: The Paradigms Framing the Future of Digital Healthcare 144
Viraaj Gupta and B.K. Tripathy
9. Integrating IoT, Analytics and Deep Learning in ECG for Cardiovascular care 166
Tuhin Mukherjee

10. Transfer Learning for Multiclass Classification of Bone Marrow Cells 184
Rishabh Hanselia, Dilip Kumar Choubey, Kanchan Bala and Ashutosh Mishra

Index 217

CHAPTER

1

Machine Learning and the Role of IoT in Health Informatics

Burak TAŞCI*

Firat University Vocational School of Technical Sciences, 23119, Elazig, Turkey

The innovations brought by Industry 4.0 to health informatics and the challenges encountered are discussed. Industry 4.0 initiates a new era in the healthcare sector through the integration of technologies like IoT, machine learning, cloud computing, and big data analytics. These technological advancements have enabled healthcare services to become more efficient, personalized, and accessible. Particularly, the use of IoT sensors that monitor various health parameters such as heart rate, blood pressure, and glucose levels, has facilitated continuous health tracking and enhanced early diagnosis opportunities, marking significant innovations of this era. However, challenges such as data security, privacy, and ethical issues brought by these technological developments are also considered. Accessibility and justice issues highlight the importance of technological advancements providing equal opportunities for all. This book chapter comprehensively examines the impacts of Industry 4.0 on health informatics, addressing future trends and potential developments in this field. It underscores how this innovative era enhances the quality of healthcare services while also bringing new challenges to the forefront.

1. Introduction

Industrial development commenced in the 18th century with the discovery of steam power, marking the first phase of technological advancement. The turn of the 19th and 20th centuries saw the onset of the Industry 2.0 era, characterized by the widespread use of electrical power and the evolution of mass production

*Corresponding author: Btasci@firat.edu.tr

methodologies. In the second half of the 20th century, the development of computerization and automation systems initiated a new epoch, referred to as Industry 3.0. The dawn of the 21st century heralded the Industry 4.0 era, driven by innovations such as the Internet of Things (IoT), artificial intelligence, cloud computing, big data analytics, cyber-physical systems, simulation, RFID technologies, and advanced robotics. The Industry 4.0 era is defined by reduced human intervention and increased automation. During this period, technologies like machine-to-machine communication (M2M) and IoT enable unique global interactions over the internet among objects, revolutionizing various industrial and commercial sectors [1, 2].

Health informatics, as a field aimed at enhancing the quality, efficiency, and accessibility of healthcare services, has become a fundamental component of Industry 4.0 [3-5]. Technologies such as electronic health records, clinical information systems, and telehealth applications enable more effective monitoring of patients' health conditions and optimization of treatment processes. The integration of machine learning and IoT has expanded the potential of health informatics and reshaped the future of healthcare services. Machine learning plays a crucial role in the early diagnosis of diseases and the development of personalized treatment plans. On the other hand, IoT facilitates communication between physical devices over the internet and with central systems, contributing to more proactive and patient-centered healthcare services.

In this section, we examine the impact of Industry 4.0 on health informatics and how this technological transformation is shaping the future of healthcare services [6, 7]. The intersection of machine learning and IoT technologies is driving digital transformation in the healthcare sector, enabling innovative applications that enhance patients' quality of life. These developments not only improve the quality and accessibility of healthcare services but also bring to the forefront the challenges and ethical issues encountered. In today's world, the use of information and communication technologies in the delivery of healthcare services is widespread. This has laid the foundation for the emergence of health informatics, a discipline that denotes the use of information technologies in the health sector. The advancements in the field of health informatics encompass the following evolutionary stages [8]:

- Transition from Analog to Digital Recording Systems: The shift from paper-based data recording methods to computer-supported digital recording systems.
- Evolution from Departmental to Comprehensive Information Systems: Moving beyond simple departmental recording systems to integrated information systems at the hospital or healthcare institution level, and then to regional health information systems.
- Increased User Diversity: In health informatics systems, not only healthcare institution staff but also patients and other individuals have become active users.

- Utilization of Health Data for Various Purposes: Health data are used not only for treatment and administrative needs but also for planning and clinical research.
- Diversification of Data Types: In addition to numerical data, the processing of medical images and molecular data has become feasible.
- Use of Sensor Technologies: The use of sensor technologies in the data collection process of health informatics systems has gained importance.

The Internet of Things (IoT) is a network of technologies that enables physical devices, vehicles, home appliances, and other objects to communicate with each other and with larger systems over the internet. This technology allows objects to collect data, analyze it, and turn it into action through sensors, software, and other technologies. In the healthcare sector, the combined use of machine learning and IoT technologies can significantly improve patient care and treatment methods.

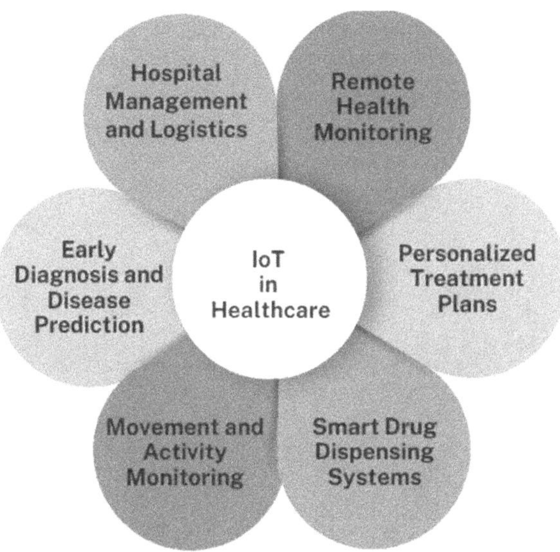

Figure 1. IoT areas in health

IoT devices can continuously monitor patients' health conditions at home. Examples include heart rate monitors, blood pressure meters, and glucose monitors. The data from these devices, when analyzed by machine learning algorithms, can detect abnormal conditions and send alerts to healthcare professionals [9].

Remote Health Monitoring: IoT devices enable the ongoing monitoring of patients' health conditions from their homes. Devices such as heart rate monitors, blood pressure meters, and glucose monitors provide data that, when analyzed by machine learning algorithms, can identify abnormal conditions and trigger alerts to healthcare professionals.

Personalized Treatment Plans: Machine learning can analyze large datasets to create treatment plans personalized to a patient's condition. Data from IoT devices reflect the patient's current state, allowing for continuous updates to their treatment plans [10, 11].

Smart Drug Dispensing Systems: IoT-based smart medication dispensers can monitor patients' medication adherence. Machine learning can develop reminders and alerts to enhance patient compliance [12, 13].

Movement and Activity Monitoring: Wearable devices and sensors can track patients' physical activities and movements. This data can be used to monitor the rehabilitation process and accelerate the recovery journey [14, 15].

Early Diagnosis and Disease Prediction: Continuous health data collected from IoT devices, analyzed through machine learning algorithms, can be utilized for early diagnosis of diseases and identification of risk factors [16, 17].

Hospital Management and Logistics: IoT sensors can be employed in managing hospital resources, such as bed occupancy and medical equipment status. Machine learning analyses this data to optimize resource allocation [18-20].

This book chapter will focus on Remote Health Monitoring and the sensors employed in this innovative field.

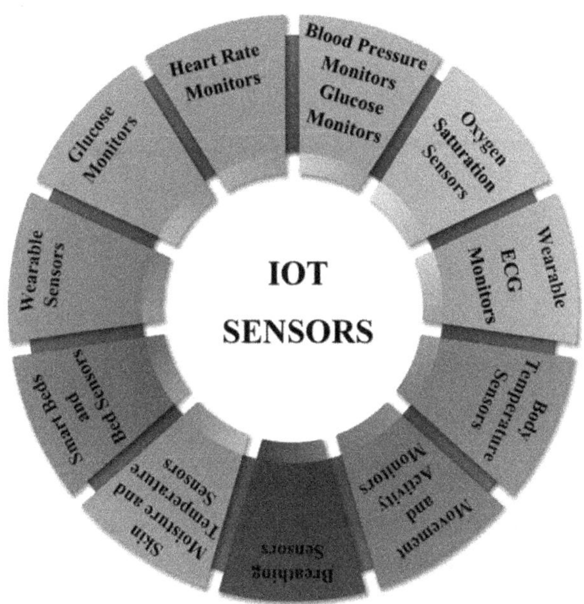

Figure 2. IoT sensor types

IoT sensors for continuous health monitoring encompass a wide range and aid in improving patient care by tracking various health parameters. In the literature, disease detection is made using EEG [21, 22], ECG [23] signals, X-ray [24],

OCT [25], computed tomography and MRI [26-28] images. Below are some commonly used IoT sensors in this field, described for clarity.

Heart Rate Monitors: Heart rate monitors are biomedical devices playing a critical role in measuring and monitoring cardiac functions. These devices have the capability to detect each heartbeat and continuously record the heart rate. Their basic working principle involves recording the heart's electrical activity and expressing this data as heart rate. Traditionally, these devices utilize electrocardiogram (ECG)-based methods. An ECG records the heart's electrical activity through electrodes placed on the skin surface. These electrodes detect electrical changes with each heartbeat and process this information to calculate the heart rate [29]. In recent years, wearable heart rate monitors developed using optical sensor technology have also gained popularity. Typically in the form of a wristband or smartwatch, these devices detect changes in blood flow beneath the skin using the photoplethysmogram (PPG) method. PPG measures the impact of changes in blood volume under the skin on light absorption or reflection and uses this information to calculate heart rate [30]. The use of heart rate monitors is significant in both clinical and personal health monitoring. In clinical settings, these devices are used for continuous monitoring of patients' cardiovascular status, while in personal use, they serve as an effective tool for tracking physical activity, sports performance, and overall health assessment. These technologies hold great potential for monitoring heart health and developing early warning systems. However, issues such as the accuracy of devices, wearability comfort, and privacy of user data remain significant focus areas for research and development in this field [31].

Blood Pressure Monitors: Blood pressure monitors are medical devices of critical importance in monitoring cardiovascular health. These devices measure arterial blood pressure, providing essential information about hemodynamic status [32]. Blood pressure contains crucial information about the heart's pumping function and the state of the arterial system and consists of two main components. Systolic Pressure is the pressure during the heart's contraction (systole) phase, when blood is pushed into the arteries at the highest pressure [33]. Diastolic Pressure is the moment during the heart's relaxation (diastole) phase, when the pressure in the arteries is at its lowest [34, 35]. Blood pressure monitors are primarily found in two types. Manual Blood Pressure Monitors typically include a cuff, stethoscope, and sphygmomanometer. This method, used by health professionals, is based on listening to Korotkoff sounds. The cuff is wrapped around the user's arm and inflated until arterial blood flow stops. Then, as the pressure is gradually released, Korotkoff sounds are listened to via the stethoscope, and the points where these sounds start and stop are recorded as the systolic and diastolic pressures. Digital Blood Pressure Monitors automatically inflate the cuff and measure blood pressure via a sensor, displaying results on digital screens that are easy to read. These devices are ideal for home blood pressure monitoring, offering users a more practical and quicker measurement option. The accuracy and reliability of blood pressure monitors are closely related to the device's quality, correct usage, and regular calibration. Especially for hypertension management and early diagnosis of cardiovascular diseases, these devices are considered fundamental tools. However, factors such as patient position, cuff size, and placement during the use of these devices are critical in ensuring the accuracy of the measurements [36, 37].

Glucose Monitors: Glucose monitors are biomedical devices used for measuring glucose (sugar) levels in the blood [38]. Playing a central role in diabetes management, these devices enable patients to regularly monitor their glucose levels, aiming to maintain blood sugar within an appropriate range and reduce the risks of hypoglycemia or hyperglycemia. The primary function of glucose monitors is to measure the amount of glucose in a small blood sample. Some advanced glucose monitors developed today are known as Continuous Glucose Monitoring systems (CGM) and use less invasive methods. CGMs typically measure glucose levels in the interstitial fluid continuously through a small sensor placed under the skin. These sensors transmit glucose readings wirelessly to a receiver or smartphone at regular intervals, allowing users to track their real-time glucose values and their variations over time [39]. The accuracy of glucose monitors is critical for the effectiveness of diabetes management [40]. Accurate and consistent results from these devices are essential for effectively managing blood sugar and reducing the risk of complications associated with diabetes. Proper use of the device by users, appropriate storage of test strips, and regular calibration of the device enhance the reliability of the measurements.

Oxygen Saturation Sensors (Pulse Oximeters): Oxygen Saturation Sensors, commonly known as "pulse oximeters," are medical devices that measure blood oxygen saturation (SpO2) and heart rate [41]. These devices are primarily used for assessing respiratory functions and monitoring the general oxygenation status. SpO2 represents the percentage of arterial blood saturated with oxygen, typically ranging between 95-100% in healthy individuals. Pulse oximeters typically operate with a probe placed on the finger, earlobe, or the bridge of the nose. Their fundamental principle is based on the differential absorption of light of different wavelengths by oxygenated and deoxygenated blood. The device emits light at two different wavelengths (usually red and infrared) into the bloodstream. Oxygenated and deoxygenated hemoglobin absorb these lights at different rates. The device calculates the blood oxygen saturation level by detecting the amount of transmitted light. This method is non-invasive (the device does not need to enter the body) and offers continuous, real-time monitoring. Pulse oximeters are critically important in managing respiratory diseases, heart failure, patient monitoring in intensive care units, and during anesthesia [42]. The accuracy of pulse oximeters can be affected by factors such as skin pigmentation, circulatory disorders, movement, external light sources, and the type of probe used [36, 41]. The use of these devices effectively monitors oxygenation status in clinical and home settings and assists in the early detection of potentially life-threatening conditions. However, understanding the limitations of pulse oximeters and interpreting their data within the context of a comprehensive clinical assessment is important.

Wearable EKG Monitors: Wearable ECG (Electrocardiogram) monitors are devices designed to continuously or periodically monitor the electrical activity of the heart. These devices combine the functionality provided by traditional ECG machines with wearable technology, offering users greater mobility and comfort [43]. They are used for the early detection and monitoring of cardiac arrhythmias, ischemia (insufficient blood flow to the heart), and other cardiovascular diseases. Wearable ECG monitors typically include electrodes, a data processing unit, and a data transmission system. The electrodes are placed on the skin and detect the heart's electrical activity. These signals are analyzed by the processing unit and are often wirelessly transmitted to a smartphone or computer. One of the primary advantages of these devices is the ability to offer prolonged and continuous monitoring. Users can record cardiac activity while continuing with their daily activities, which is particularly important for detecting intermittent arrhythmias that may not be captured by traditional, short-term ECG recordings. Wearable ECG devices are also used in telemedicine and remote patient monitoring applications [44, 45]. These devices transmit patients' cardiac data in real time to healthcare providers, enabling remote monitoring and intervention. This feature has become particularly important during and after the pandemic. The accuracy and reliability of these technologies depend on factors such as the quality of electrode-skin contact, motion artifacts, and environmental influences. Furthermore, the interpretation of data provided by these devices requires professional medical knowledge, and the results should typically be evaluated by a health professional. Wearable ECG monitors are considered a significant innovation in the field of cardiovascular health monitoring, and ongoing technological advancements in this area will further enhance the effectiveness and usability of these devices [46, 47].

Body Temperature Sensors: Body temperature sensors are biomedical devices used to measure the core and surface temperatures of the human body. These devices play a critical role in health assessment, particularly in detecting conditions such as infections and inflammation [48, 49]. Body temperature is considered an indicator of metabolic and physiological processes and is a significant marker of health status. Body temperature sensors can be of various types and use different measurement methods:

Contact-Based Sensors: These sensors measure temperature through direct contact with the skin. Traditional mercury thermometers, digital thermometers, and ear thermometers fall into this category. These devices generally provide accurate and reliable measurements, but correct usage is essential for accurate results [50, 51].

Non-contact (Contactless) Sensors: Devices such as infrared thermometers and thermal cameras detect body temperature by measuring infrared radiation emitted from the skin's surface. Their contactless nature allows for quick and hygienic measurements, though environmental factors and device calibration can affect measurement accuracy [50].

Wearable Sensors: Recent advancements in wearable technology have significantly impacted body temperature sensors. Wearable devices such as smartwatches, fitness bands, and smart textiles can provide continuous body temperature monitoring [52]. These devices enable users to monitor their health status while continuing their daily activities. The use of body temperature sensors is important in clinical and home settings for patient monitoring, fever detection, and general health assessment. Particularly, these sensors are critical tools for the early detection of infectious diseases and inflammatory conditions [53-55]. The effectiveness of these devices depends on correct usage, regular calibration, and interpretation of measurement results from a professional health perspective [56, 57].

Movement and Activity Monitors: Movement and Activity Monitors are devices designed to measure and record individuals' physical activities and movement levels. These devices are used to monitor daily activities, exercises, and overall mobility, providing critical data for physical health and lifestyle analysis [14]. These monitors typically include sensors that record parameters such as the number of steps, distance covered, calories burned, exercise duration, and sometimes even sleep quality. Advanced models can also measure more complex metrics like altitude climbed, heart rate, body temperature, and even stress levels. The use of movement and activity monitors can help increase physical activity levels, achieve health and fitness goals, and monitor overall health status [58]. Especially effective in managing chronic diseases, rehabilitation processes, and promoting a healthy lifestyle, these technologies can boost users' motivation and support healthy behavior changes [59, 60]. However, the accuracy of movement and activity data depends on the device's quality and usage conditions, and the interpretation of this data in line with health and fitness goals is essential.

Respiration Sensors: Respiration Sensors are devices that measure and analyze individuals' breathing patterns, respiratory rates, and volumes [61]. These devices are used for assessing respiratory functions, detecting respiratory disorders, and monitoring overall health status. Respiration sensors are used in various areas, including clinical settings for personal health monitoring and during sports training. They are employed for evaluating respiratory functions, diagnosing and monitoring respiratory disorders (such as asthma and COPD), detecting breathing pauses during sleep and assessing sleep quality, and evaluating athletes' and fitness enthusiasts' breathing patterns and performance. Breathing patterns are closely related to stress levels, and these sensors can be used to monitor the effectiveness of stress management and relaxation techniques. The use of respiration sensors enables comprehensive monitoring of respiratory health and assists in the early detection of potential health issues [62, 63]. These devices can be especially vital for individuals with chronic respiratory diseases. However, accurate interpretation of data provided by these sensors and its integration with professional medical assessment is crucial. With technological advancements, respiration sensors are becoming more advanced and hold a significant place in personal health monitoring.

Skin Moisture and Temperature Sensors: Moisture Sensors measure the amount of moisture on the skin, typically through changes in the skin's electrical conductivity or capacitance. As the skin's moisture level increases, electrical conductivity usually rises [64]. Temperature Sensors measure the skin surface's temperature, which can be done using thermistors or infrared sensors. Thermistors operate on the principle of resistance change with temperature variations, while infrared sensors measure infrared radiation emitted from the skin. Skin moisture and temperature sensors are used in various areas. They are utilized for diagnosing and monitoring skin health and diseases. For instance, monitoring skin moisture is important in conditions like eczema or psoriasis. They help determine skin type and assist in selecting appropriate skincare products. They are used to understand the relationship between skin moisture and temperature, and various dermatological and systemic diseases. They are employed for monitoring athletes' thermoregulation and hydration status [65]. In chronic disease management and elderly care, they can be used for remote monitoring of skin health [66, 67]. Skin Moisture and Temperature Sensors are non-invasive and typically wearable devices, allowing users to monitor skin health continuously without interrupting daily life. The accuracy of these sensors depends on the device's quality, skin contact, and environmental factors. For a comprehensive assessment of skin health, it is important to combine the data from these sensors with dermatological expertise and other health information. Technological advancements are making these sensors more sensitive, user-friendly, and widely available.

Smart Beds and Bed Sensors: Smart Beds and Bed Sensors are technological devices used to monitor, improve, and manage sleep quality and various health conditions related to sleep. These devices help track individuals' sleep quality and overall health status by measuring parameters such as body movements, sleep positions, respiratory rhythm, heart rate, and sometimes body temperature during sleep [68, 69]. Smart beds and bed sensors are used in various areas. They track parameters like sleep duration, time to fall asleep, sleep stages, and awakenings throughout the night. They are used in managing sleep apnea, chronic pain, and other sleep-related health conditions [70].They monitor movements and health status of individuals who spend prolonged periods in bed and can also be effective in preventing bedsores. Some smart beds can adjust features like firmness and temperature according to the needs during sleep.

Smart beds and bed sensors continuously and non-invasively monitor physiological and behavioral parameters during sleep, helping to improve sleep quality and overall health status. These technologies provide valuable information to health professionals about patients' conditions and assist individuals in improving their sleep habits. However, the correct interpretation of data from these devices and evaluation from a professional health perspective is important. With technological advancements, smart beds and bed sensors are becoming increasingly sophisticated and hold a significant place in personal health monitoring and home care services [71, 72].

2. Machine Learning and IoT

The convergence of Machine Learning (ML) and the Internet of Things (IoT) forms a significant area of interest in today's technological world [73-79]. The primary goal of integrating these two fields is to process the large streams of data from IoT devices and extract more meaningful and useful information. Primarily, machine learning provides the ability to learn from large and complex datasets, which is vital for analyzing raw data (e.g., sensor data) collected by IoT devices and deriving beneficial insights. Machine learning models can use these data to identify patterns, detect abnormal behaviors, and predict future trends.

The continuous data generation by IoT devices necessitates their immediate processing and analysis. Machine learning aids in this process by efficiently processing data, thereby enhancing the performance, security, and efficiency of IoT systems. This is particularly critical for real-time applications. Overall, the amalgamation of machine learning and IoT aims to create a more connected and efficient technological environment by enabling smarter use of data. This integration allows for maximizing the use of data collected by IoT devices, with machine learning algorithms effectively processing this data to offer new and valuable insights. This synergy significantly contributes to the technological advancements of the future, enabling smarter and more autonomous functioning of devices both in our homes and industrial applications. In the literature, there are various artificial intelligence techniques [80-82] and IoT applications. Some of these are tabulated in Table 1.

These sensors, by providing real-time data, enable continuous monitoring of patients' health conditions, thereby increasing the opportunities for early intervention. With the advancement of technology, more sophisticated and diverse health monitoring sensors are being developed and utilized.

3. Conclusion

This book chapter thoroughly examines the impact of Industry 4.0 on health informatics, highlighting how technologies like IoT and machine learning are transforming healthcare services. Industry 4.0 has been a pioneer in the digitalization and automation of the healthcare sector, leading to significant advancements in patient care and treatment methods. Particularly, the integration of IoT devices and machine learning algorithms has contributed to making healthcare services more proactive, personalized, and accessible. This transformation is supported by the development of various IoT sensors such as

Table 1. IoT and artificial intelligence applications in literature

Ref	Year	Sensor/Data Type	Methods	Result (%)
Chorba et al. [83]	2021	Digital stethoscope	CNN	Sensitivity: 93.20 Specificity: 86.00
Gómez-Quintana et al. [84]	2021	Digital stethoscope	Segmentation, Feature Extraction, XGBoost	AUC: 78.00
Tiwari et al. [85]	2021	Phonocardiogram Signal	Mel Frequency Cepstral, Chroma Energy Normalized Statistics, and Constant-Q Transform	Accuracy: 96.00
González et al. [86]	2023	Photoplethysmogram	Fast Fourier transform, Naive Bayes 5 Fold Cross Validation	Mean absolute scaled error: 100
Ali et al. [87]	2023	Photoplethysmogram	LSTM-ANN	Mean absolute error: 1.41
Rodríguez-Rodríguez et al. [88]	2023	Continuous glucose monitoring	PSW, Lasso	Root mean square error: 98.43
Boonnag et al .[89]	2023	Pulse Oximeter	YOLOv4, YOLOv5, YOLOR	Accuracy: 81.0–89.5
Khanna et al .[90]	2023	Wearable ECG Monitors	IoT and deep learning (DL) enabled healthcare disease diagnosis (IoTDL-HDD) model	Accuracy: 93.45

heart rate monitors, blood pressure, and glucose monitors. These devices have played crucial roles in continuous health monitoring and the development of early warning systems. Furthermore, machine learning has become a critical factor in early disease diagnosis and the development of personalized treatment plans through big data analysis. However, these technological advancements also bring new challenges. Data privacy, security, and ethical issues are among the most pressing concerns in this field. Additionally, the accessibility and usability of technology can be significant barriers to providing equal healthcare services for all. Therefore, along with technological innovations, the societal and ethical aspects of these technologies must also be considered. In conclusion, the effects of Industry 4.0 on health informatics present both significant opportunities and serious challenges. This new era, while shaping the future of healthcare services, must also consider societal and ethical responsibilities. This balanced approach will ensure the delivery of more effective, accessible, and equitable healthcare services and lay the foundation for future innovations.

References

[1] Alam, M., Nielsen, R.H. and Prasad, N.R. The evolution of M2M into IoT. 2013 First International Black Sea Conference on Communications and Networking (BlackSeaCom): IEEE, 112-115, 2013.

[2] Shah, S.H. and Yaqoob, I. A survey: Internet of Things (IOT) technologies, applications and challenges. 2016 IEEE Smart Energy Grid Engineering (SEGE), 381-385, 2016.

[3] Zhang, C. and Chen, Y. A review of research relevant to the emerging industry trends: Industry 4.0, IoT, blockchain, and business analytics. Journal of Industrial Integration and Management, 5: 165-180, 2020.

[4] Okano, M.T. IOT and industry 4.0: The industrial new revolution. International Conference on Management and Information Systems, 26, 2017.

[5] Manavalan, E. and Jayakrishna, K. A review of Internet of Things (IoT) embedded sustainable supply chain for industry 4.0 requirements. Computers & Industrial Engineering, 127: 925-953, 2019.

[6] Cheng, G.-J., Liu, L.-T., Qiang, X.-J. and Liu, Y. Industry 4.0 development and application of intelligent manufacturing. 2016 International Conference on Information System and Artificial Intelligence (ISAI): IEEE, 407-410, 2016.

[7] Karboub, K., Tabaa, M., Dandache, A., Dellagi, S. and Moutaouakkil, F. Toward health 4.0: Challenges and opportunities. International Conference on Innovation and New Trends in Information Technology, 20-21, 2019.

[8] Haux, R. Health information systems – Past, present, future. International Journal of Medical Informatics, 75: 268-281, 2006.

[9] Majumder, S., Mondal, T., Deen, M.J. Wearable sensors for remote health monitoring. Sensors, 17: 130, 2017.

[10] Pitts, N. and Richards, D. Personalized treatment planning. Detection, Assessment, Diagnosis and Monitoring of Caries, 21: 128-143, 2009.

[11] Sheth, A., Jaimini, U. and Yip, H.Y. How will the internet of things enable augmented personalized health? IEEE Intelligent Systems, 33: 89-97, 2018.
[12] Kumar, N., Kaushal, R.K. and Panda, S.N. IoT based smart and portable system for remote patient monitoring and drug delivery. Journal of Physics: Conference Series: IOP Publishing, 012017, 2021.
[13] Raikar, A.S., Kumar, P., Raikar, G.S. and Somnache, S.N. Advances and challenges in IoT-based smart drug delivery systems: A comprehensive review. Applied System Innovation, 6: 62, 2023.
[14] Bisio, I., Delfino, A., Lavagetto, F. and Sciarrone, A. Enabling IoT for in-home rehabilitation: Accelerometer signals classification methods for activity and movement recognition. IEEE Internet of Things Journal, 4: 135-146, 2016.
[15] Mighali, V., Patrono, L., Stefanizzi, M.L., Rodrigues, J.J., Solic, P. et al. A smart remote elderly monitoring system based on IoT technologies. 2017 Ninth International Conference on Ubiquitous and Future Networks (ICUFN): IEEE, 43-48, 2017.
[16] Kumar, P.M., Lokesh, S., Varatharajan, R., Babu, G.C., Parthasarathy, P. et al. Cloud and IoT based disease prediction and diagnosis system for healthcare using Fuzzy neural classifier. Future Generation Computer Systems, 86: 527-534, 2018.
[17] Muthu, B., Sivaparthipan, C., Manogaran, G., Sundarasekar, R., Kadry, S. et al. IOT based wearable sensor for diseases prediction and symptom analysis in healthcare sector. Peer-to-peer Networking and Applications. 13: 2123-2134, 2020.
[18] Rico, J., Cendón, B., Lanza, J. and Valiño, J. Bringing IoT to hospital logistics systems demonstrating the concept. 2012 IEEE Wireless Communications and Networking Conference Workshops (WCNCW): IEEE, 196-201, 2012.
[19] Guo, J. and Yang, J. An IOT-based hospital logistics management system. International Conference on Intelligent Systems, Communications, and Computer Networks (ISCCN 2023): SPIE, 68-75, 2023.
[20] Thamrongaphichartkul, K., Worrasittichai, N., Prayongrak, T. and Vongbunyong, S. A framework of IoT platform for autonomous mobile robot in hospital logistics applications. 2020 15th International Joint Symposium on Artificial Intelligence and Natural Language Processing (iSAI-NLP): IEEE, 1-6, 2020.
[21] Tasci, I., Tasci, B., Barua, P.D., Dogan, S., Tuncer, T. et al. Epilepsy detection in 121 patient populations using hypercube pattern from EEG signals. Information Fusion, 96: 252-268, 2023.
[22] Tasci, G., Gun, M.V., Keles, T., Tasci, B., Barua, P.D. et al. QLBP: Dynamic patterns-based feature extraction functions for automatic detection of mental health and cognitive conditions using EEG signals. Chaos, Solitons & Fractals, 172: 113472, 2023.
[23] Tasci, B., Tasci, G., Dogan, S. and Tuncer, T. A novel ternary pattern-based automatic psychiatric disorders classification using ECG signals. Cognitive Neurodynamics, 1-14, 2022.
[24] Taşci, B. Deep Learning-based approaches using feature selection methods for automatic diagnosis of COVID-19 disease from X-ray images. Deep Learning Applications in Image Analysis, Springer. 27-50, 2023.
[25] Arslan, S., Kaya, M.K., Tasci, B., Kaya, S., Tasci, G. et al. Attention TurkerNeXt: Investigations into bipolar disorder detection using OCT images. Diagnostics, 13: 3422, 2023.

[26] Tatli, S., Macin, G., Tasci, I., Tasci, B., Barua, P.D. et al. Transfer-transfer model with MSNet: An automated accurate multiple sclerosis and myelitis detection system. Expert Systems with Applications, 236: 121314, 2024.

[27] Ekmekyapar, T. and Taşcı, B. Exemplar MobileNetV2-based artificial intelligence for robust and accurate diagnosis of multiple sclerosis. Diagnostics, 13: 3030, 2023.

[28] Tas, N.P., Kaya, O., Macin, G., Tasci, B., Dogan, S. et al. ASNET: A novel AI framework for accurate ankylosing spondylitis diagnosis from MRI. Biomedicines, 11: 2441, 2023.

[29] Chhabra, M. and Kalsi, M. Real time ECG monitoring system based on Internet of Things (IoT). International Journal of Scientific and Research Publications. 7: 547-550, 2017.

[30] Dinh, A., Luu, L. and Cao, T. Blood pressure measurement using finger ECG and photoplethysmogram for IoT. 6th International Conference on the Development of Biomedical Engineering in Vietnam (BME6) 6: Springer. 83-89, 2018.

[31] Abel, J.D.K., Dhanalakshmi, S., Sanjana, N. and Kumar, R. IoT-based heart rate monitoring system for smart healthcare applications. Intelligent and Soft Computing Systems for Green Energy, 273-285, 2023.

[32] Lamonaca, F., Balestrieri, E., Tudosa, I., Picariello, F., Carnì, D.L. et al. An overview on Internet of medical things in blood pressure monitoring. 2019 IEEE International Symposium on Medical Measurements and Applications (MeMeA): IEEE, 1-6, 2019.

[33] Jahan, I., Rahman, M.L., Reza, A.W. and Barman, S.D. Systolic blood pressure measurement from heart rate using IoT. International Journal of Recent Technology and Engineering (IJRTE), 7: 135-138, 2018.

[34] Pardeshi, V., Sagar, S., Murmurwar, S. and Hage, P. Health monitoring systems using IoT and Raspberry Pi—A review. 2017 International Conference on Innovative Mechanisms for Industry Applications (ICIMIA): IEEE, 134-137, 2017.

[35] Saji, M., Sridhar, M., Rajasekaran, A., Kumar, R.A., Suyampulingam, A. et al. Iot-based intelligent healthcare module. Advances in Smart System Technologies: Select Proceedings of ICFSST 2019. Springer. 765-774, 2021.

[36] Sangeethalakshmi, K., Preethi, U. and Pavithra, S. Patient health monitoring system using IoT. Materials Today: Proceedings, 80: 2228-2231, 2023.

[37] Namkoong, M., Baskar, B., Singh, L., Guo, H., McMurray, J. et al. Add-on soft electronic interfaces for continuous cuffless blood pressure monitoring. Advanced Materials Technologies, 2300158, 2023.

[38] Gia, T.N., Ali, M., Dhaou, I.B., Rahmani, A.M., Westerlund, T. et al. IoT-based continuous glucose monitoring system: A feasibility study. Procedia Computer Science, 109: 327-334, 2017.

[39] Vashist, S.K. Continuous glucose monitoring systems: A review. Diagnostics, 3: 385-412, 2013.

[40] Rahmat, M.A., Su, E., Addi, M.M. and Yeong, C. GluQo: IoT-based non-invasive blood glucose monitoring. Journal of Telecommunication, Electronic and Computer Engineering (JTEC), 9: 71-75, 2017.

[41] Murali, D., Rao, D.R., Rao, S.R. and Ananda M. Pulse oximetry and IOT based cardiac monitoring integrated alert system. 2018 International Conference on Advances in Computing, Communications and informatics (ICACCI): IEEE, 2237-2243, 2018.

[42] Nookala Venu, D., Kumar, A. and Rao, M. Internet of Things based pulse oximeter for health monitoring system. NeuroQuantology, 20: 5056-5066, 2022.

[43] Yang, Z., Zhou, Q., Lei, L., Zheng, K., Xiang, W. et al. An IoT-cloud based wearable ECG monitoring system for smart healthcare. Journal of Medical Systems, 40: 1-11, 2016.

[44] Spanò, E., Di Pascoli, S. and Iannaccone, G. Low-power wearable ECG monitoring system for multiple-patient remote monitoring. IEEE Sensors Journal, 16: 5452-5462, 2016.

[45] Azariadi, D., Tsoutsouras, V., Xydis, S. and Soudris, D. ECG signal analysis and arrhythmia detection on IoT wearable medical devices. 2016 5th International Conference on Modern Circuits and Systems Technologies (MOCAST): IEEE, 1-4, 2016.

[46] John, A., Padinjarathala, A., Doheny, E., Cardiff, B., John, D. et al. An evaluation of ECG data fusion algorithms for wearable IoT sensors. Information Fusion, 96: 237-251, 2023.

[47] Sadad, T., Safran, M., Khan, I., Alfarhood, S., Khan, R. et al. Efficient classification of ECG images using a lightweight CNN with attention module and IoT. Sensors, 23: 7697, 2023.

[48] Zakaria, N.A., Saleh, F.N.B.M. and Razak, M.A.A. IoT (Internet of Things) based infant body temperature monitoring. 2018 2nd International Conference on Biosignal Analysis, Processing and Systems (ICBAPS): IEEE, 148-153, 2018.

[49] Nookhao, S., Thananant, V. and Khunkhao, T. Development of IoT heartbeat and body temperature monitoring system for community health volunteer. 2020 Joint International Conference on Digital Arts, Media and Technology with ECTI Northern Section Conference on Electrical, Electronics, Computer and Telecommunications Engineering (ECTI DAMT & NCON): IEEE, 106-109, 2020.

[50] Hoang, M.L., Carratù, M., Paciello, V. and Pietrosanto, A. Body temperature—Indoor condition monitor and activity recognition by mems accelerometer based on IoT-alert system for people in quarantine due to COVID-19. Sensors, 21: 2313, 2021.

[51] KP, D., Martin, N. and KS, S. Iot based contactless body temperature measurement and data collection for covid 19. Proceedings of the International Conference on IoT Based Control Networks & Intelligent Systems-ICICNIS 2021.

[52] Stavropoulos, T.G., Papastergiou, A., Mpaltadoros, L., Nikolopoulos, S., Kompatsiaris, I. et al. IoT wearable sensors and devices in elderly care: A literature review. Sensors, 20: 2826, 2020.

[53] Singh, K.R., Nayak, V., Singh, J. and Singh, R.P. Nano-enabled wearable sensors for the Internet of Things (IoT). Materials Letters, 304: 130614, 2021.

[54] De Fazio, R., De Vittorio, M. and Visconti, P. Innovative IoT solutions and wearable sensing systems for monitoring human biophysical parameters: A review. Electronics, 10: 1660, 2021.

[55] Mamdiwar, S.D., Shakruwala, Z., Chadha, U., Srinivasan, K., Chang, C.-Y. et al. Recent advances on IoT-assisted wearable sensor systems for healthcare monitoring. Biosensors, 11: 372, 2021.

[56] Costanzo, A., Augello, E., Battistini, G., Benassi, F., Masotti, D. et al. Microwave devices for wearable sensors and IoT. Sensors, 23: 4356, 2023.

[57] Talaat, F.M. and El-Balka, R.M. Stress monitoring using wearable sensors: IoT techniques in medical field. Neural Computing and Applications, 1-14, 2023.

[58] Qi, J., Yang, P., Waraich, A., Deng, Z., Zhao, Y. et al . Examining sensor-based physical activity recognition and monitoring for healthcare using Internet of Things: A systematic review. Journal of Biomedical Informatics, 87: 138-153, 2018.

[59] Faliagka, E., Skarmintzos, V., Panagiotou, C., Syrimpeis, V., Antonopoulos, C.P. et al. Leveraging edge computing ML model implementation and IoT paradigm towards reliable postoperative rehabilitation monitoring. Electronics. 12: 3375, 2023.

[60] Subhan, F., Mirza, A., Su'ud, M.B.M., Alam, M.M., Nisar, S. et al. AI-enabled wearable medical internet of things in healthcare system: A survey. Applied Sciences, 13: 1394, 2023.

[61] del Bosque, A., Sánchez-Romate, X.F., Patrizi, D., del Río Sáez, J.S., Wang, D.-Y. et al. Ultrasensitive flexible strain sensors based on graphene nanoplatelets doped poly (ethylene glycol) diglycidyl ether: Mask breathing monitoring for the Internet of Things. Sensors and Actuators A: Physical, 358: 114448, 2023.

[62] Tiele, A., Wicaksono, A., Ayyala, S.K. and Covington, J.A. Development of a compact, IoT-enabled electronic nose for breath analysis. Electronics, 9: 84, 2020.

[63] Raji, A., Devi, P.K., Jeyaseeli, P.G. and Balaganesh, N. Respiratory monitoring system for asthma patients based on IoT. 2016 Online International Conference on Green Engineering and Technologies (IC-GET): IEEE, 1-6, 2016.

[64] Li, W.D., Ke, K., Jia, J., Pu, J.H., Zhao, X., Bao, R.Y. et al. Recent advances in multiresponsive flexible sensors towards E-skin: A delicate design for versatile sensing. Small, 18: 2103734, 2022.

[65] Hariharakrishnan, J. and Bhalaji, N. Adaptability analysis of 6LoWPAN and RPL for healthcare applications of Internet-of-Things. Journal of ISMAC, 3: 69-81, 2021.

[66] Kabiri Ameri, S., Ho, R., Jang, H., Tao, L., Wang, Y., Wang, L. et al. Graphene electronic tattoo sensors. ACS Nano, 11: 7634-7641, 2017.

[67] Fang, Y., Chen, G., Bick, M. and Chen, J. Smart textiles for personalized thermoregulation. Chemical Society Reviews. 50: 9357-9374, 2021.

[68] García-Magariño, I., Lacuesta, R. and Lloret, J. Agent-based simulation of smart beds with internet-of-things for exploring big data analytics. IEEE Access, 6: 366-379, 2017.

[69] Elsokah, M.M. and Zerek, A.R. Next generation of medical care bed with internet of things solutions. 2019 19th International Conference on Sciences and Techniques of Automatic Control and Computer Engineering (STA): IEEE, 84-89, 2019.

[70] Hong, Y.-S. Smart care beds for elderly patients with impaired mobility. Wireless Communications and Mobile Computing, 2018, 2018.

[71] Maddeh, M., Hajjej, F., Alazzam, M.B., Otaibi, S.A., Turki, N.A. and Ayouni, S. Spatio-temporal cluster mapping system in smart beds for patient monitoring. Sensors, 23: 4614, 2023.

[72] Tak, S.H., Choi, H., Lee, D., Song, Y.A. and Park J. Nurses' perceptions about smart beds in hospitals. Computers, Informatics, Nursing, 41: 394, 2023.

[73] Thakur, D., Saini, J.K. and Srinivasan, S. DeepThink IoT: The strength of deep learning in Internet of Things. Artificial Intelligence Review, 1-68, 2023.

[74] Mishra, S. and Tyagi, A.K. The role of machine learning techniques in Internet of Things-based cloud applications. Artificial Intelligence-based Internet of Things Systems, 105-135, 2022.

[75] Tahsien, S.M., Karimipour, H. and Spachos, P. Machine learning based solutions for security of Internet of Things (IoT): A survey. Journal of Network and Computer Applications, 161: 102630, 2020.

[76] Bose, A., Roy, S.S., Balas, V.E. and Samui, P. Deep learning for brain computer interfaces. Handbook of Deep Learning Applications, 333-344, 2019.

[77] Roy, S.S. and Taguchi, Y.-H. Identification of genes associated with altered gene expression and m6A profiles during hypoxia using tensor decomposition based unsupervised feature extraction. Scientific Reports, 11: 8909, 2021.
[78] Basu, A., Roy, S.S. and Abraham, A. A novel diagnostic approach based on support vector machine with linear kernel for classifying the erythemato-squamous disease. 2015 International Conference on Computing Communication Control and Automation: IEEE, 343-347, 2015.
[79] Pandey, A.K. and Roy, S.S. Natural language generation using sequential models: A survey. Neural Processing Letters, 1-34, 2023.
[80] Roy, S.S., Roy, A., Samui, P., Gandomi, M. and Gandomi, A.H. Hateful sentiment detection in real-time tweets: An LSTM-based comparative approach. IEEE Transactions on Computational Social Systems, 2023.
[81] Roy, S.S., Pratyush, C. and Barna, C. Predicting ozone layer concentration using multivariate adaptive regression splines, random forest and classification and regression tree. Soft Computing Applications: Proceedings of the 7th International Workshop Soft Computing Applications (SOFA 2016), Volume 27: Springer, 140-152, 2018.
[82] Roy, S.S., Gupta, A., Sinha, A. and Ramesh, R. Cancer data investigation using variable precision rough set with flexible classification. Proceedings of the Second International Conference on Computational Science, Engineering and Information Technology, 472-475, 2012.
[83] Chorba, J.S., Shapiro, A.M., Le, L., Maidens, J., Prince, J., Pham, S. et al. Deep learning algorithm for automated cardiac murmur detection via a digital stethoscope platform. Journal of the American Heart Association, 10: e019905, 2021.
[84] Gómez-Quintana, S., Schwarz, C.E., Shelevytsky, I., Shelevytska, V., Semenova, O., Factor, A. et al. A framework for AI-assisted detection of patent ductus arteriosus from neonatal phonocardiogram. Healthcare: MDPI, 169, 2021.
[85] Tiwari, S., Jain, A., Sharma, A.K. and Almustafa, K.M. Phonocardiogram signal based multi-class cardiac diagnostic decision support system. IEEE Access, 9: 110710-110722, 2021.
[86] González, S., Hsieh, W.-T. and Chen, T.P.-C. A benchmark for machine-learning based non-invasive blood pressure estimation using photoplethysmogram. Scientific Data, 10: 149, 2023.
[87] Ali, N.F. and Atef, M. An efficient hybrid LSTM-ANN joint classification-regression model for PPG based blood pressure monitoring. Biomedical Signal Processing and Control, 84: 104782, 2023.
[88] Rodríguez-Rodríguez, I., Campo-Valera, M., Rodríguez, J.-V. and Frisa-Rubio, A. Constrained IoT-based machine learning for accurate glycemia forecasting in type 1 diabetes patients. Sensors. 23: 3665, 2023.
[89] Boonnag, C., Ittichaiwong, P., Saengmolee, W., Seesawad, N., Chinkamol, A., Rattanasomrerk, S. et al. PACMAN: A framework for pulse oximeter digit detection and reading in a low-resource setting. IEEE Internet of Things Journal, 2023.
[90] Khanna, A., Selvaraj, P., Gupta, D., Sheikh, T.H., Pareek, P.K., Shankar, V. Internet of things and deep learning enabled healthcare disease diagnosis using biomedical electrocardiogram signals. Expert Systems, 40: e12864, 2023.

CHAPTER

2

Bioconductor Packages to Perform Tensor Decomposition Based Unsupervised Feature Extraction

Y-h. Taguchi*

Chuo University, Tokyo, Japan

TDbasedUFE and TDbasedUFEadv are recently developed Bioconductor package by which people can apply tensor decomposition based unsupervised feature extraction to their own data set without the knowledge about tensor decomposition. In this chapter, we introduce these two packages with some applications.

1. Introduction

Tensor decomposition (TD) based unsupervised feature extraction (TD) was proposed a few years ago [1]. In spite of the successful application of TD based unsupervised FE to genomic science, it remained unpopular possibly because of the unpopularity of tensor decomposition. We have recently developed two bioconductor packages, TDbasedUFE and TDbasedUFEadv [2], to allow researchers without knowledge about tensor decomposition to make use of TD based unsupervised FE. In this chapter, we introduce how people can make use of these packages to use TD based unsupervised FE.

2. TDbasedUFE

TDbasedUFE is a primary package to perform TD based unsupervised FE. It concentrates on two most popular features of TD based unsupervised FE, i.e., identification of differentially expressed genes (DEGs) and multiomics analysis.

---

*Corresponding author: tag@granular.com

2.1 Single Omics — Gene Expression Profiles

For DEG identification, gene expression is typically formatted as a tensor $x_{ijk} = \sum_{\ell_1=1}^{N}\sum_{\ell_2=1}^{M}\sum_{\ell_3=1}^{K} G(\ell_1\ell_2\ell_3)u_{\ell_i i}u_{\ell_2 j}u_{\ell_3 k}$ which represents the expression of the ith gene of the jth sample at the kth condition. HOSVD is applied to x_{ijk} and we get

$$x_{ijk} = \sum_{\ell_1=1}^{N}\sum_{\ell_2=1}^{M}\sum_{\ell_3=1}^{K} G(\ell_1\ell_2\ell_3)u_{\ell_i i}u_{\ell_2 j}u_{\ell_3 k} \tag{1}$$

In TD based unsupervised FE, it is important to identify which singular value vectors (SVVs) attributed to samples or experimental conditions, i.e., $u_{\ell_2 j}$ and $u_{\ell_3 k}$ are of interest. For example, if samples, js, corresponds to distinction between patients (j = 1) and healthy control (j = 2), the selected ℓ_2 should be associated with $u_{\ell_2 1} = -u_{\ell_2 2}$. On the other hand, if the kth condition corresponds to simply the kth biological replicate, $u_{\ell_3 k}$ is better with a constant value regardless of k.

In TDbasedUFE, this selection of ℓ_2 and ℓ_3 are provided to users by graphical user interfase (GUI). Then selected ℓ_2 and ℓ_3 are forwarded for downstream analysis. All things that users must do other than selecting SVVs attributed to samples or experimental conditions is to re-format gene expression profiles usually provided in a matrix format to tensor format, which can be easily done by the dim command. Suppose that the object x is a $N \times M$ matrix and we would like to have the tensor of the dimension $N \times M/K \times K$. This can be done in R by dim(x) <– c(N,M/K,N).

To demonstrate TDbasedUFE, we have employed gene expression profiles deposited at GEO with GEO ID GSE212759 [3]. We have also downloaded the file "GSE212759_Lyn_lck_normalised_counts.txt.gz". It is composed of six samples grouped into three groups, each of which is composed of two biological replicates. Three groups are composed of control, over expression of Lck and Lyn genes. The number of genes whose expression is measured is N = 47,388. Then gene expression profiles are formatted as $x_{ijk} \in \mathbb{R}^{N \times 2 \times 3}$ that represents the expression of the ith gene at the jth biological replicates of the kth experimental condition (j = 1 control, j = 2 Lck over expression, and j = 3 Lyn over expression). At first, we need to select which ℓ_2 attributed to biological replicates and which ℓ_3 attributed to conditions of interest (see eq. (1)). Since $u_{\ell_2 j}$ attributed to biological replicates should take constant values regardless of j, we need to find which $u_{\ell_2 j}$ take constant values, i.e. $u_{\ell_2 1} = u_{\ell_2 2}$. Then we found that ℓ_2 = 1 satisfied this requirement; it is very usual the first singular value vectors take constant values regardless of the considered problem. Next we need to find which $u_{\ell_3 k}$ is distinct between K = 1 and $k \neq 1$ since the former is control and the latter is treated sample. Then we found that ℓ_3 = 2 is associated with this requirement. These selections must be performed by visual inspection in GUI that TDbasedUFE provides. All things we have to do is only selection of ℓ_2 and is, and find 4,259 is associated with adjusted P-values less than 0.01. These genes are uploaded by the enrichr function in the packages enrichR as described in Enrichment vignettes in TDbasedUFEadv. Specifically, we consider three categories, "GO Molecular Function 2023" (GO MF), "GO Cellular Component 2023" (GO CC), and "GO Biological Process 2023" (GI MF). Then we found that 292, 93 and 63 terms are associated with adjusted P-values less than 0.05. Although this does not always mean that the analyses were successful, since they cannot be successful if there are no enriched terms. Atleast the existence of terms associated with significant P-values is a necessary condition for success. Figure 1 shows the top ranked terms graphically. Since these are translation related terms and we tried to identify differentially expressed genes, our analyses seemed to be successful.

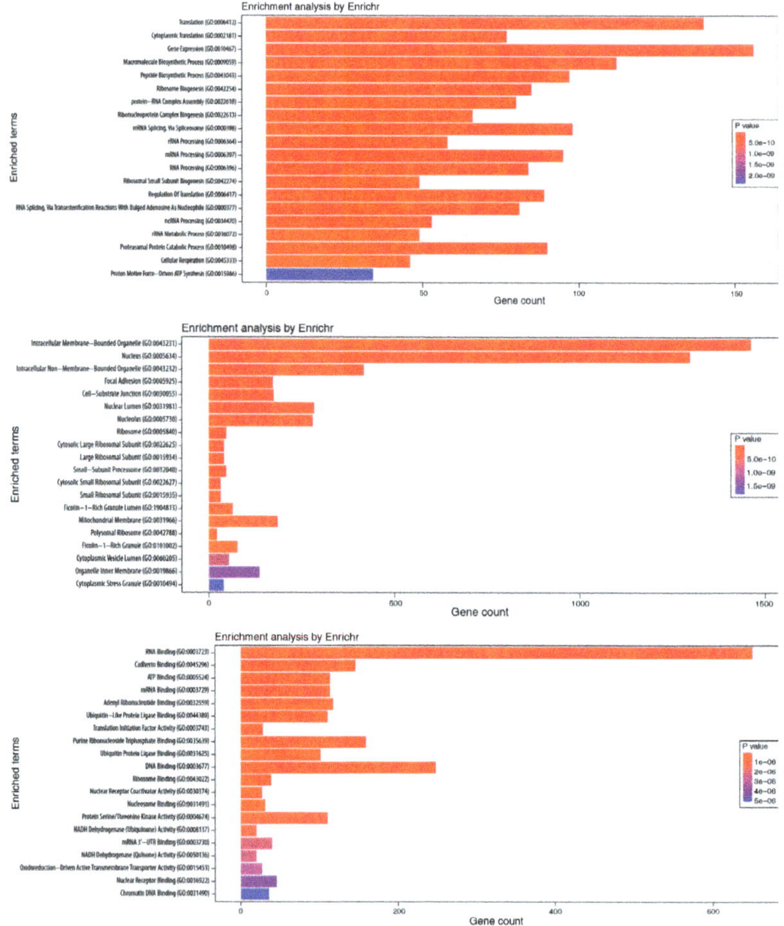

Figure 1. Enrichment analyses: top, GO BP, middle, GO CC, bottom, GO MF

2.2 Multiomincs Analysis

Next, we tried to use the second function implemented in TDbasedUFE, i.e., multiomics analyses. To do this, we employed a data set retrieved from GEO with GEO ID GSE210392 [4], which is composed of two GEO data sets, GSE210390 and GSE210391. From GSE210390, we downloaded GSE210390_SCI_RNAseq rawCounts.xlsx from Supplementary file section for gene expression profile and GSE210391_RAW.tar from GSE210391 that included 32 methylation profiles. Gene expression profiles and DNA methylation profiles share 32 samples as shown in Table 1.

Table 1. Number of samples with individual conditions. SCI: Spinal cord injury

		Spinal Cord Injury	
Days after treatment	**Control**	**Vehicle**	**Boldine**
7 days	4	6	6
28 days	4	6	6

These profiles are formatted as a tensor $x_{i_k jk} \in \mathbb{R}^{N_k \times 16 \times 4}$ that represents gene expression (for $k = 1, 2$) or DNA methylation (for $k = 3, 4$) of the jth condition ($1 \leq j \leq 4$ control, $5 \leq j \leq 10$, Vehicle, $11 \leq j \leq 16$ Boldine) on the 7th day ($k = 1, 3$) and 28 days ($k = 2, 4$) after the treatment, i.e., SCI. Although $N_1 = N_2 = 55{,}487$ is the number of genes, since N_3 and N_4 are the numbers of methylation sites, N_3 or N_4 differ from $N_1 = N_2$. At first, we list all the methylation sites, which are as many as 10,111,999, that appear at least once in 32 samples shown in Table 1. Then missing values are filled with 0. To make a tensor from $x_{i_k jk}$, we compute their self-product as

$$z_{jj'k} = \sum_{i_k=1}^{N_k} x_{i_k jk} x_{i_k j'k} \in \mathbb{R}^{16 \times 16 \times 4} \tag{2}$$

to which HOSVD was applied after the normalization

$$\sum_{j=1}^{16} \sum_{j=1'}^{16} z_{jj'k} = 16^2 \tag{3}$$

and we get

$$z_{jj'k} = \sum_{\ell_1=1}^{16} \sum_{\ell_2=1}^{16} \sum_{\ell_3=1}^{4} G(\ell_1 \ell_2 \ell_3) u_{\ell_1 j} u_{\ell_2 j'} u_{\ell_3 k} \tag{4}$$

where $G \in \mathbb{R}^{16 \times 16 \times 4}$ is the core tensor, $u_{\ell_1 j}, u_{\ell_2 j'} \in \mathbb{R}^{16 \times 16}$, $u_{\ell_3 k} \in \mathbb{R}^{4 \times 4}$ are singular value and orthogonal matrices. At first, we need to identify which $u_{\ell_2 j'}$ and $u_{\ell_3 k}$ are associated with desired properties; $u_{\ell_2 1}$ attributed to control should be distinct from $u_{\ell_2 2}$ and $u_{\ell_2 2}$ attributed to treated samples whereas $u_{\ell_3 1}$ and $u_{\ell_3 2}$ attributed to gene expression are distinct from $u_{\ell_3 3}$ and $u_{\ell_3 4}$ attributed to methylation (if possible, it is better to be associated with opposite signs).

TDbasedUFE allows users to select ℓ_2 and ℓ_3 with GUI and we selected $\ell_2 = 3$ and $\ell_3 = 4$, respectively by visual inspection. After that, TDbasedUFE automatically selected 4,089 i_1s, 2,788 i_2s, 386,096 i_3s and 637,620 i_4s. Since i_1 and i_2 are represented as an ensemble mouse gene ID, 4,089 and 2,788 ensemble mouse gene IDs are converted to 4,025 and 2,724 gene symbols with select function using org.Mm.eg.db [5]. These gene symbols are uploaded to Enrichr with **enrichr** function as well and we got enrichment results for GO BP, GO CC and GO MF. The number of enriched terms are 764, 177, and 143 for $k = 1$ (seven days after treatment) and 594,83, and 79 for $k = 2$ (28 days after treatment). Since these numbers are large enough, we can conclude that the analyses is successful. Figures 2 and 3 show top ranked terms.

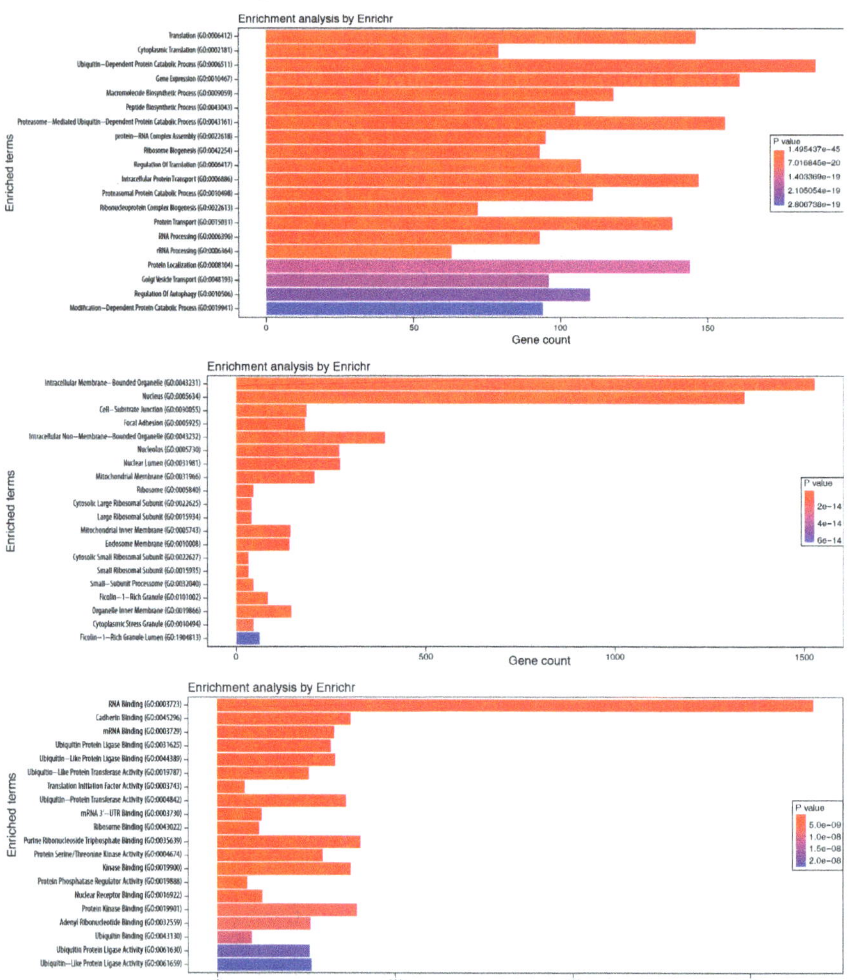

Figure 2. Enrichment analyses for $k = 1$, gene expression, seven days after treatment: top, GO BP, middle, GO CC, bottom, GO MF

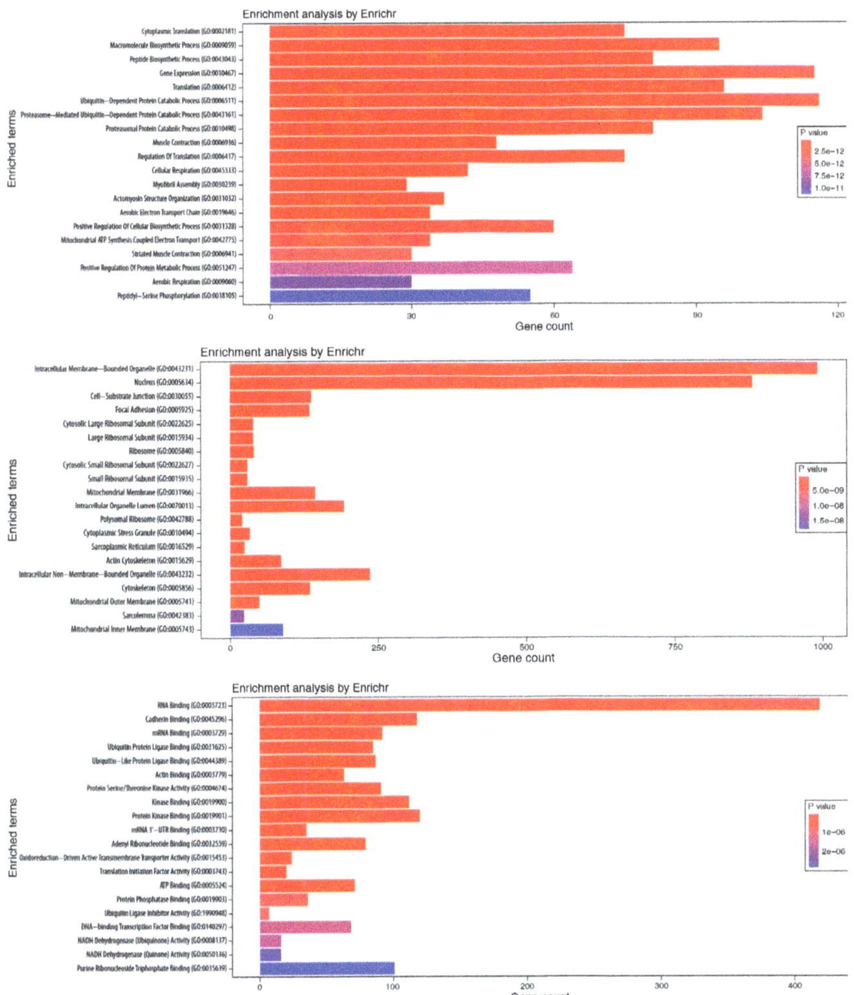

Figure 3. Enrichment analyses for $k = 2$, gene expression, 28 days after treatment: top, GO BP, middle, GO CC, bottom, GO MF.

For DNA methylation profiles, i_3s and i_4s are not genes but chromosomal locations which need to be converted to the associated gene symbols. To do this, we used annotate_regions function in annotatr [6] package in R with "mm10_genes_cds" annotation. Then we got 6,956 and 7,988 gene symbols for $k = 3$ (seven days after treatment) and $k = 4$ (28 days after treatment:), respectively. 6,956 and 7,988 gene symbols were uploaded to Enrichr with **enrichr** function. Then we got 207 GO BP terms, 45 GO CC terms and 53 GO MF terms for $k = 3$ and 236 GO BP terms, 44 GO CC terms and 56 GO MF terms for $k = 4$, respectively. Since these numbers are large enough, our analyses were successful. Figures 4 and 5 show top ranked terms.

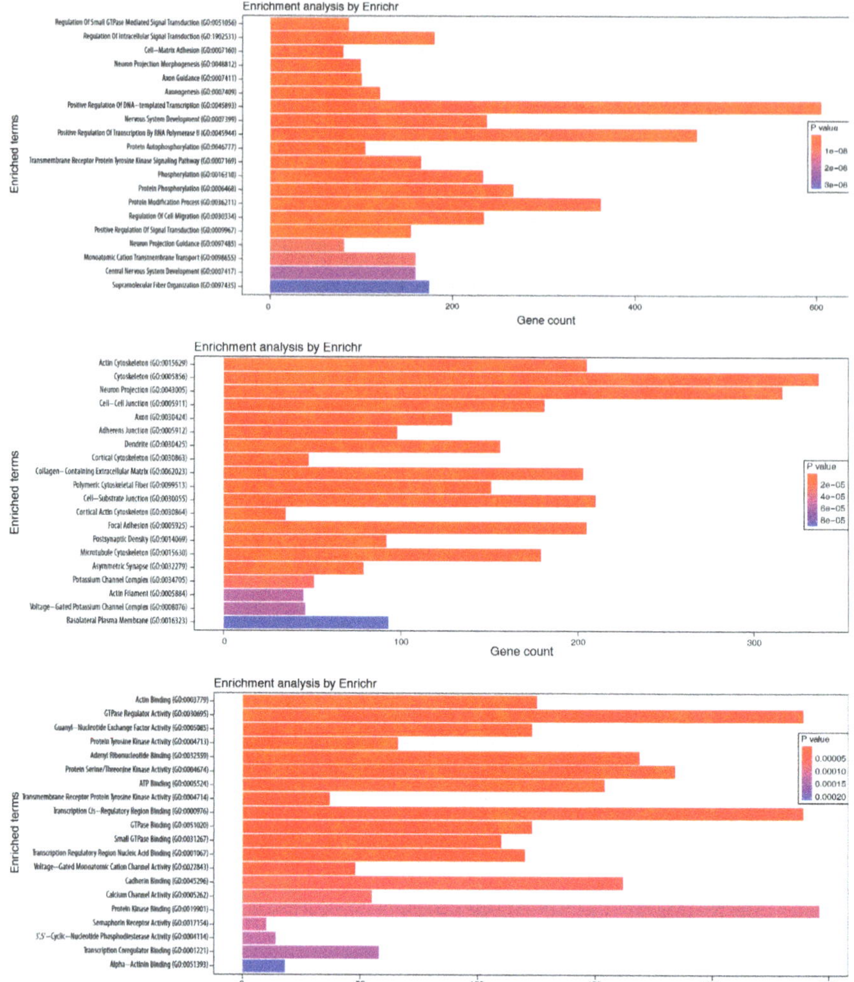

Figure 4. Enrichment analyses for $k = 3$, DNA methylation, seven days after treatment: top, GO BP, middle, GO CC, bottom, GO MF

3. TDbasedUFEadv

Next we introduce TDbasedUFEadv.

3.1 Integrated Analysis of Two Omics Data Sets that Share Features

One functionality of TDbasedUFE is to integrate two omics profiles that share features but not samples. To demonstrate this functionality, we employ two gene expression profiles $x_{i_k jk} \in \mathbb{R}^{N_k \times 16 \times 2}$, $k \leq 2$ used in the previous section. A tensor $z_{ijj'} \in \mathbb{R}^{N \times 16 \times 16}$ where $N = N_1 = N_2$ is generated as

$$z_{ijj'} = x_{ij1} x_{ij'2} \tag{5}$$

where $i = i_1 = i_2$. It is normalized as

$$\sum_{i=1}^{N} z_{ijj'} = 0, \tag{6}$$

$$\sum_{i=1}^{N} z_{ijj'}^2 = N \tag{7}$$

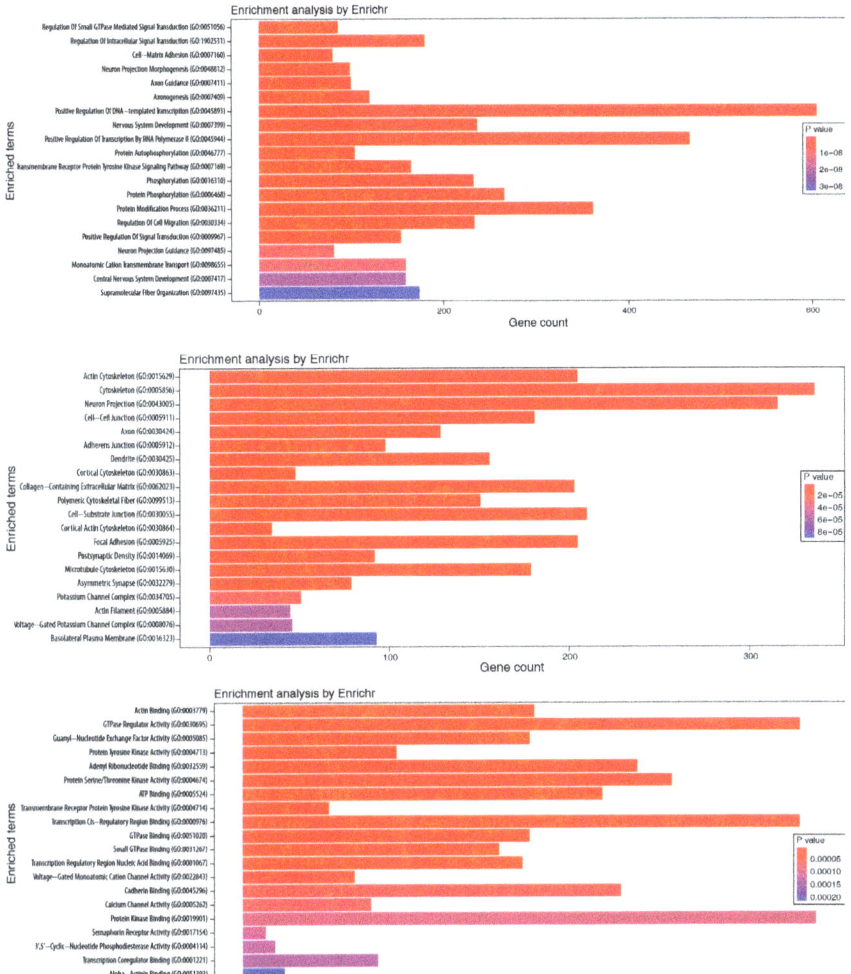

Figure 5. Enrichment analyses for $k = 4$, DNA methylation, 28 days after treatment: top, GO BP, middle, GO CC, bottom, GO MF

HOSVD is applied to $x_{ijj'}$ and we get

$$z_{ijj'} = \sum_{\ell_1=1}^{N} \sum_{\ell_2=1}^{16} \sum_{\ell_3=1}^{16} G(\ell_1 \ell_2 \ell_3) u_{\ell_1 i} u_{\ell_2 j} u_{\ell_2 j} \tag{8}$$

where $G \in \mathbb{R}^{N \times 16 \times 16}$ is the core tensor and $u_{\ell_1 i} \in \mathbb{R}^{N \times N}$, $u_{\ell_2 j}$, $u_{\ell_3 j'} \in \mathbb{R}^{16 \times 16}$ are singular value matrices and orthogonal matrices. As usual, we need to identify which $u\ell_{2j}$ and $u\ell_{3j'}$ are of interest and we found that $\ell_2 = \ell_3 = 2$ are associated with distinction between three classes, control, SCI Vehicle, and SCI Boldine (Table 1). This selection was done in TDbasedUFEadv with GUI by users. Once ℓ_2 and ℓ_3 were selected, TDbasedUFEadv automatically selects 118 is which are ensemble gene IDs. This number is substantially smaller then the number of i_1s and i_2s identified in multiomics analyses, 4,089 and 2,788 respectively. There can be multiple reasons for this small number is identified. For example, in the present analysis, since $x_{i_1 j1}$ is multiplied with $x_{i_2 j2}$, is have j dependencies for both $k = 1$ (seven days after treatment) and $k = 2$ (28 days after treatment). Thus, is identified become smaller than the individual analyses of i_1 and i_2.

After 118 gene symbols were associated with 187 is as in the previous section, 118 gene symbols were uploaded as in the previous section. Then we identified 100 GO BP terms, 34 GO CC terms, and 27 GO MF terms. Although these numbers are also smaller than those in multiomics analysis, they are large enough for considering the analysis to be successful. Figure 6 shows the list of top ranked enriched terms.

3.2 Reduction of Required Memory Using Partial Summation

When features are shared, we can reduce memory requirements by summation of i as

$$z_{jj'} = \sum_{i=1}^{N} z_{ijj'} \in \mathbb{R}^{16 \times 16} \tag{9}$$

SVD is applied to $z_{jj'}$ and we got

$$z_{jj'} = \sum_{\ell=1}^{L} \lambda_{\ell u_{\ell j} u_{\ell j'}} \tag{10}$$

As usual, we need to identify which $u_{\ell j}$ and $v_{\ell j'}$ are of interest. Those of interest should be distinct between three classes, control, SCI Vehicle, and SCI Boldine (Table 1). Then we found that $\ell = 2$ satisfies this requirement (This selection can be done with GUI in TDbasedUFEadv). Missing SVVs attributed to i_1 and i_2 can be recovered as

$$u_{\ell i1} = \sum_{j=1}^{16} x_{i_1 j1} u_{\ell j} \tag{11}$$

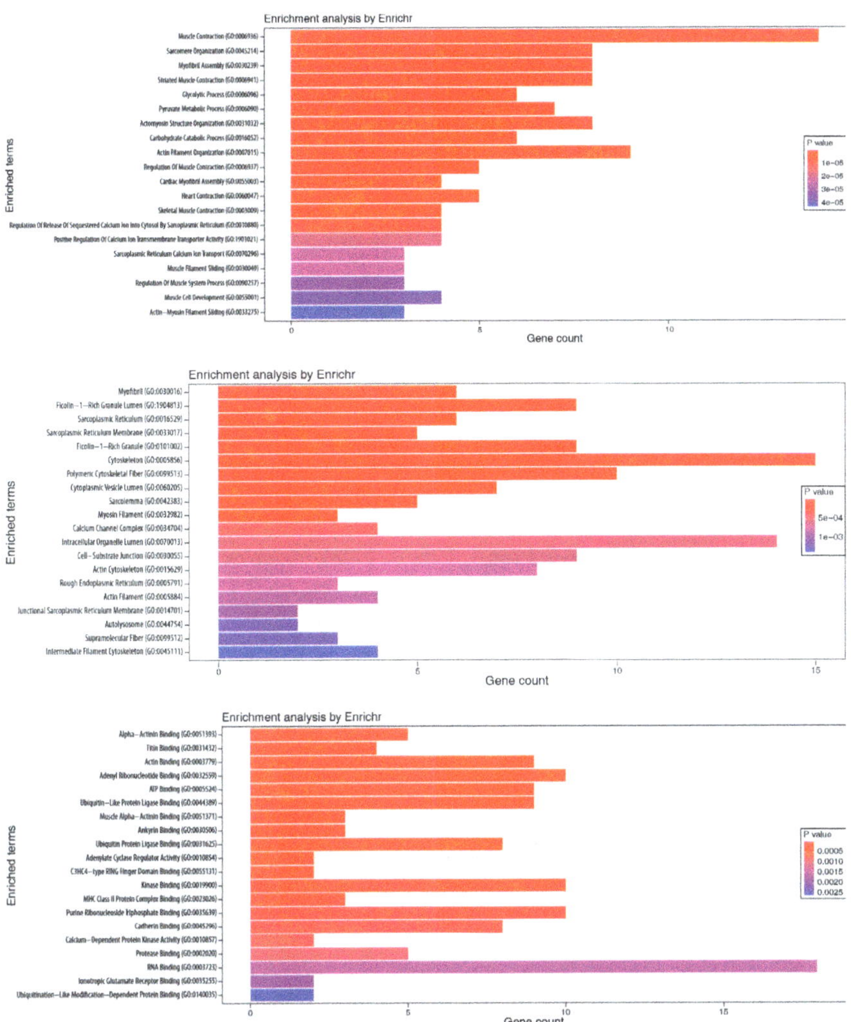

Figure 6. Enrichment analyses for integrated analysis of two gene expression profiles, top, GO BP, middle, GO CC, bottom, GO MF

$$u_{\ell i 2} = \sum_{j'=1}^{16} x_{i_2 j' 2} u_{\ell j} \tag{12}$$

and 2,440 i_1s and 2,403 i_2s were automatically selected based upon P-values attributed to $u_{\ell i1}$ and $u_{\ell i2}$ within TDbasedUFEadv. Since the requirement of coincidence between i_1 (seven days after treatment) and i_2 (28 days after treatment) is less, we can have more number of i_1s and i_2s compared with the previous section where only one set of *i*s was selected commonly between i_1s and i_2s. 2,419 and 2,352 gene symbols associated with the i_1s and i_2s are identified, respectively, as above and uploaded to Enrichr as above. Then we got 597 GO BP terms, 135 GO CC terms, and 111 GO MF terms for i_1 (seven days after treatment) and 431 GO BP terms, 89 GO CC terms, and 76 GO MF terms for i_2 (28 days after treatment). Since these numbers are large enough, our analyses was successful. Figures 7 and 8 show top ranked GO terms.

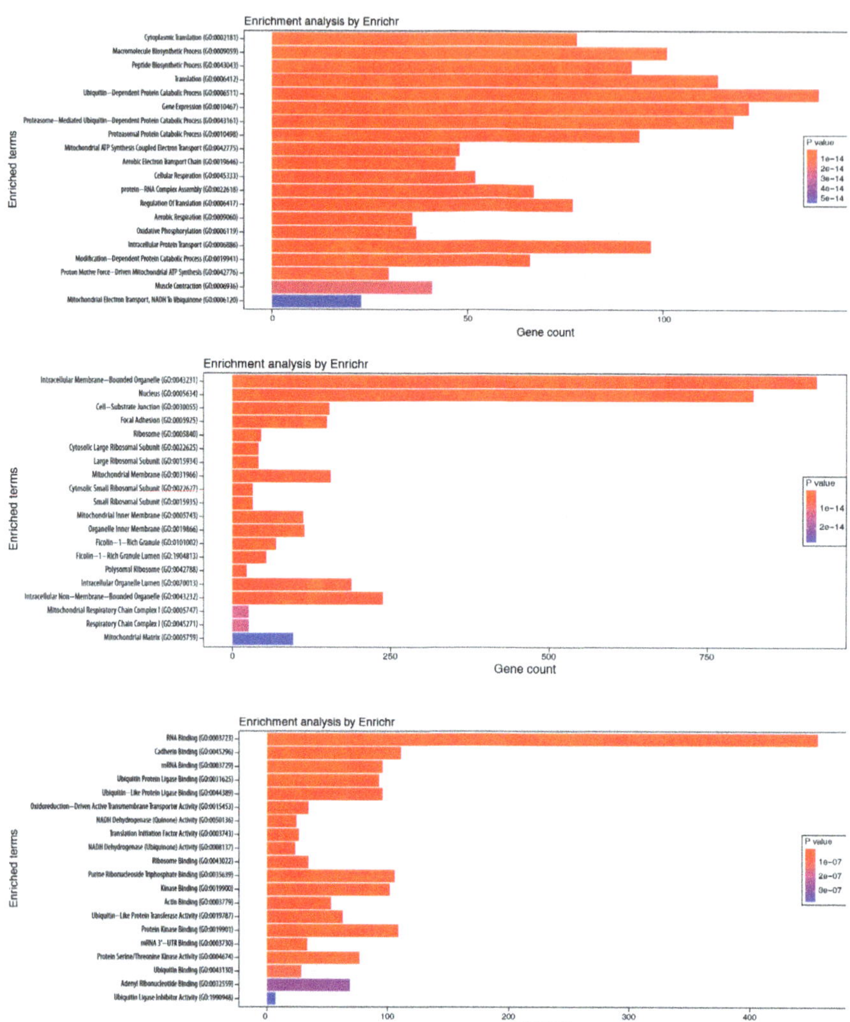

Figure 7. Enrichment analyses for $k = 1$, gene expression, seven days after treatment: top, GO BP, middle, GO CC, bottom, GO MF, by integrated analysis

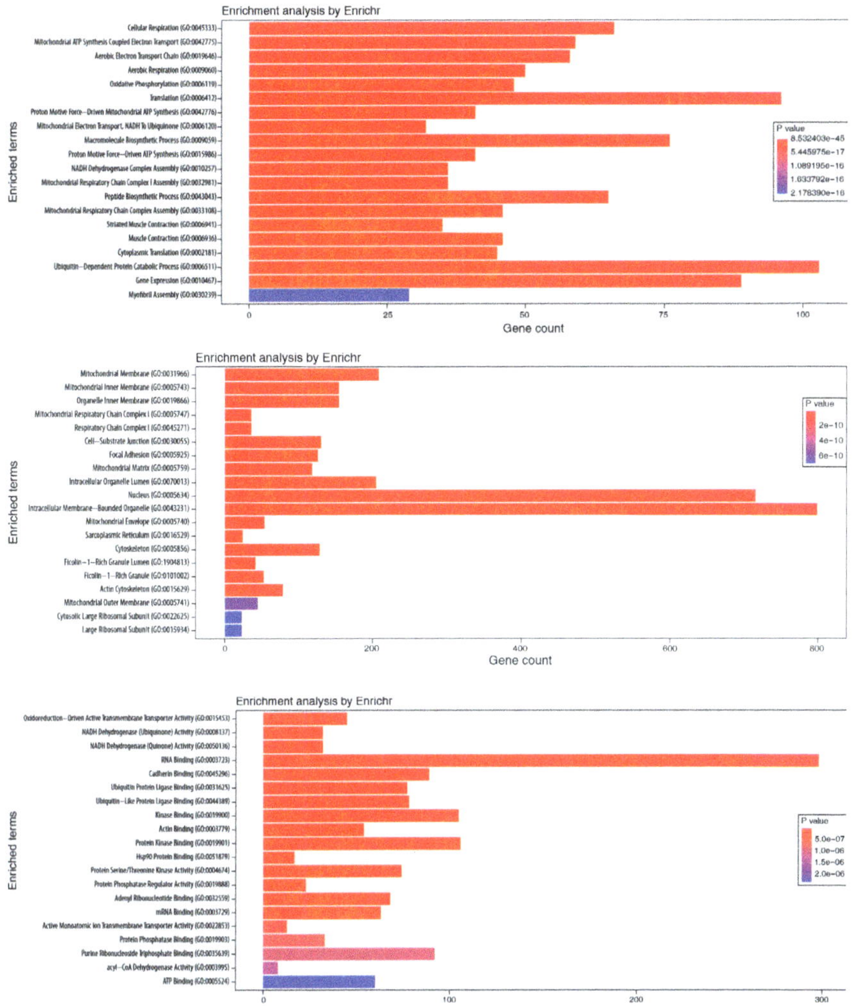

Figure 8. Enrichment analyses for $k = 1$, gene expression, seven days after treatment: top, GO BP, middle, GO CC, bottom, GO MF, by integrated analysis

4. Conclusions

In this chapter, we introduced the usage of two bioconductor packages recently developed. Although we could not introduce all the features in this chapter, since they have well documented vigettes, one can make use of these packages for this purpose as well.

References

[1] Taguchi, Y-h. Unsupervised Feature extraction Applied to Bioinformatics: A PCA-based and TD-based Approach. Springer, 2020.

[2] Taguchi, Y-h. and Turki Turki. Application note: Tdbasedufe and tdbasedufeadv: Bioconductor packages to perform tensor decomposition based unsupervised feature extraction. Frontiers in Artificial Intelligence, 6, 2023.

[3] Nikolaos Koutras, Vasileios Morfos, Kyriakos Konnaris, Adamantia Kouvela. Integrated signaling and transcriptome analysis reveals SRC family kinase individualities and novel pathways controlled by their constitutive activity. Frontiers in Immunology, 14, 2023.

[4] Luke A. Potter, Carlos A. Toro, Lauren Harlow, Kaleen M. Lavin, Christopher P. Cardozo et al. Assessing the impact of boldine on the gastrocnemius using multiomics profiling at 7 and 28 days post-complete spinal cord injury in young male mice. Physiological Genomics, 55(7): 297–313, 2023. PMID: 37125768.

[5] Marc Carlson. org.Mm.eg.db: Genome wide annotation for Mouse, 2023. R package version 3.17.0, https://doi.org/doi:10.18129/B9.bioc.org.Mm.eg.db.

[6] Raymond G. Cavalcante and Maureen A. Sartor. Annotatr: Genomic regions in context. Bioinformatics, 2017. R package version 1.26.0, https://doi.org/doi:10.18129/B9.bioc.annotatr.

CHAPTER

3

Smart Health: Advancements in Machine Learning and the Internet of Things Solutions

Narasimha Rao Vajjhala[1*][0000-0002-8260-2392] **and Philip Eappen**[2][0000-0002-8120-8449]

[1] Faculty of Engineering and Architecture, University of New York Tirana, Tirana, Albania

[2] School of Business, Cape Breton University, Cape Breton, Canada

This chapter examines the transformative intersection of healthcare analytics, Machine Learning (ML), and the Internet of Things (IoT), exploring how these state-of-the-art technologies reshape healthcare delivery. This chapter focuses on the benefits brought about by the synergy of ML and IoT in the healthcare sector, such as enhanced patient care, early disease detection, operational efficiency, and personalized treatment plans. We explore the problems and challenges of integrating ML and IoT with healthcare analytics and recommend solutions in this chapter. It also addresses ethical, practical, and security considerations, emphasizing the importance of data privacy, model interpretability, bias mitigation, and secure connectivity in deploying healthcare technology. Furthermore, this chapter also presents the ongoing technological advancements and their potential to augment healthcare analytics further, emphasizing the need for patient-centric approaches and addressing global health disparities. This chapter explores healthcare analytics' current landscape and prospects, considering the integration of ML and IoT solutions.

1. Introduction

The integration of healthcare, ML, and the IoT represents a revolutionary shift in healthcare delivery and management [1]. This integration allows for more

*Corresponding author: narasimharao@unyt.edu.al

personalized, efficient, and predictive healthcare, reshaping the landscape of health services and influencing patient outcomes, provider practices, and healthcare costs. IoT devices facilitate real-time monitoring of patients' vital signs, reducing the need for hospitalization [2]. ML algorithms analyse the data to detect anomalies and predict potential health issues, enabling timely interventions and reducing complications [3]. ML algorithms offer tailored treatment plans to individual patients by analysing historical data and predicting responses to different treatments, leading to more effective and efficient healthcare outcomes [4]. ML algorithms and IoT enhance diagnostic accuracy by analysing vast datasets, detecting patterns, and predicting diseases early, thus improving the prognosis and reducing mortality rates [4, 5].

IoT facilitates better management of healthcare resources, including staff, equipment, and facilities, through real-time tracking and ML-driven demand predictions, optimizing utilization and reducing costs [6]. ML and IoT improve workflow through automation, predictive equipment maintenance, and scheduling optimization, thereby enhancing healthcare delivery, and reducing operational costs. The integration enables better tracking and prediction of supply needs, reducing waste and ensuring the availability of essential medical supplies. IoT devices allow remote monitoring of patients, providing convenience and reducing the need for hospital visits. ML analyses the data for personalized feedback, enhancing patient engagement and adherence to treatment plans [7]. The convergence allows for advanced telemedicine services, with ML algorithms supporting diagnosis and treatment recommendations and IoT enabling remote consultations and monitoring. IoT and ML-powered healthcare apps provide personalized health advice, reminders, and monitoring, enhancing patient experience and promoting healthy behaviours [4].

This chapter also discusses the concerns about the privacy and security of health data apart from other challenges resulting from this integration. Several integration challenges exist with the amalgamation of ML, IoT, and traditional healthcare systems [8]. Hence, there is a requirement for standardized protocols and interoperability solutions. There is a definite need to ensure compliance with healthcare regulations, necessitating a comprehensive understanding of the legal landscape and the development of compliant solutions. The convergence of these technologies can enhance the prediction and management of epidemics by analysing large-scale health data, enabling timely interventions.

2. Background

Traditional healthcare analytics systematically use data and quantitative methods to identify, measure, and analyse healthcare patterns and trends, primarily focusing on improving patient outcomes, operational efficiency, and reducing costs [9]. Traditional analytics typically rely on structured, historical data from electronic health records (EHRs), billing records, and other administrative datasets [10]. Traditional analytics primarily utilize descriptive analytics to summarize and interpret historical data. It helps understand past healthcare activities, identify patterns, and report on various metrics such as patient admissions, treatment outcomes, and hospital costs.

In traditional healthcare analytics, predictive analytics involving historical data to identify patterns and trends is often applied to predict patient readmissions, disease outbreaks, and utilization of healthcare services [11]. Prescriptive analytics goes a step further by recommending actions to optimize desired outcomes [12]. It might involve suggesting treatment plans or interventions to improve patient health in healthcare. Traditional analytics help identify at-risk populations and develop targeted interventions to improve health outcomes [13]. It aids in managing healthcare costs, optimizing resource utilization, and improving healthcare organizations' financial health. Traditional analytics support clinicians in making informed decisions regarding patient care by providing insights based on historical patient data.

Healthcare organizations use analytics to monitor and improve the quality of care, adhere to regulatory standards, and enhance patient satisfaction. Traditional healthcare analytics often operate in data silos, limiting the scope of analysis and integrating varied data sources [14]. It usually takes a reactive approach, focusing on addressing issues after they occur, rather than a proactive, preventive approach. Traditional analytics primarily deal with structured data and may need help incorporating unstructured data, such as clinical notes containing valuable insights. Some healthcare organizations might need more technology infrastructure or skilled personnel to leverage analytics fully.

The advent of ML in health data analysis has marked a transformative shift in healthcare, offering unprecedented capabilities in deriving insights and predicting outcomes. This development is driven by the exponential growth in healthcare data, advances in computing power, and the evolution of ML algorithms. ML models analyze historical health data to predict future events such as disease outbreaks, patient readmissions, and complications, enabling proactive interventions [15]. ML improves diagnostic accuracy by analysing complex medical images, lab results, and other clinical data, thereby enhancing early detection of diseases and reducing misdiagnoses. ML tailors' treatment plans to individual patients by analyzing genetic, clinical, and lifestyle data, optimizing therapeutic efficacy, and minimizing adverse effects. ML accelerates drug discovery by analysing biological and chemical data, predicting drug responses, and optimizing clinical trials. ML optimizes healthcare operations by automating workflows, forecasting resource needs, and reducing costs [16]. EHRs are a primary source of structured health data for ML, providing comprehensive patient information. Wearables and IoT devices generate real-time, continuous health data, enhancing the richness and diversity of data available for analysis. ML algorithms can process unstructured data, such as clinical notes and medical images, extracting valuable insights that were previously inaccessible [17]. ML facilitates data integration of diverse data sources, creating a more holistic view of patient health and improving analysis accuracy.

The emergence of the IoT in healthcare has revolutionized patient monitoring and data collection, fostered real-time connectivity and significantly enhancing healthcare delivery [18]. IoT refers to the interconnected network of devices that communicate and exchange data, offering myriad applications in healthcare, from remote monitoring to personalized medicine. IoT devices enable the continuous monitoring of patients' vital signs and health metrics remotely, reducing the need for hospital visits and admissions and enabling timely intervention. For patients with chronic conditions, IoT offers a better way to manage their health, providing real-time feedback and alerts, thus preventing complications [19]. IoT devices support aging populations by monitoring their health and safety, detecting falls, and ensuring medication adherence. IoT enables real-time health data collection, providing a more accurate and timely representation of a patient's health status, which is crucial for effective treatment. IoT collects data from various sources, from wearables to implantable devices, creating a comprehensive picture of an individual's health. Integrating IoT data with EHRs enriches patient profiles and aids healthcare providers in making informed decisions. The rise of IoT paves the way for advanced telemedicine services, enabling remote consultations, diagnosis, and treatment recommendations. Integrating IoT with ML will further enhance data analysis, predictive modelling, and personalized healthcare delivery. The continuous development of IoT will contribute to building smart healthcare infrastructures with improved efficiency, patient-centric services, and reduced costs.

3. Review of Literature

ML is a vast field with a variety of techniques and methodologies. At a high level, ML techniques can be categorized into several types based on the nature of the learning signal or feedback available to a learning system. These techniques include supervised learning, unsupervised learning, deep learning, and reinforcement learning. Supervised learning algorithms are trained on a labeled dataset, meaning the training data has both the input and correct output. The goal is to learn mapping from inputs to outputs. Unsupervised Learning algorithms are trained on data without explicit labels, seeking to find structure or relationships within the data. Reinforcement learning algorithms learn by interacting with an environment and receiving feedback through rewards or penalties.

3.1 Supervised Learning Techniques in Healthcare Analytics

Supervised learning, a subset of ML, involves training models using labeled datasets where the outcome variable (or label) is known [20]. The trained model can then make predictions on new, unseen data. Supervised learning has emerged as a pivotal tool for disease prediction, enhancing early detection, and improving patient outcomes. Supervised learning models analyze patient data to identify the early signs of diseases, enabling timely interventions and improving prognosis. These models help categorize patients based on their risk levels for various conditions, aiding in personalized healthcare strategies and resource allocation. By analyzing individual patient data, supervised learning contributes to developing customized treatment plans, optimizing therapeutic efficacy, and minimizing adverse effects. Models leverage EHRs containing a patient's medical history, lab results, and diagnostic images to predict disease risk. Supervised learning can analyze genomic data to identify genetic mutations and variations linked to disease susceptibility. Integrating lifestyle and environmental data can enhance the accuracy of disease predictions, considering a more comprehensive range of risk factors. The effectiveness of supervised learning is contingent on the availability and quality of labeled datasets, which can be challenging to obtain in healthcare. Ensuring the interpretability of complex models is crucial for clinical adoption, as healthcare professionals need to understand and trust model predictions. Using sensitive health data necessitates stringent measures to safeguard patient privacy and ensure data security.

Predictive modeling involves the use of statistical and ML techniques to identify the likelihood of future outcomes based on historical data [21]. In healthcare, predictive modeling can forecast patient health outcomes, disease progression, and potential future interventions, among other things. Hospitals aim to reduce readmission rates due to the associated high costs and potential complications for the patient [22]. By predicting which patients are at higher risk of readmission, healthcare providers can take proactive measures. They predict the likelihood of a patient developing a particular disease in the future based on their current health data and lifestyle. In critical care settings, predicting patient mortality can help healthcare providers make informed decisions about treatment options. Predicting how long a patient will stay in the hospital can aid in resource allocation and management. Caruana et al. [23] showcase the use of predictive modeling emphasizing the importance of model interpretability. Using a combination of models, they found that some traditional risk factors for pneumonia, when used in complex models, could incorrectly suggest that those conditions lowered risk. This highlighted the potential dangers of black-box models in healthcare and the need for interpretable, transparent predictive models.

Hospital readmission rates are a critical metric in healthcare, not only due to the associated costs but also because they can reflect the quality of care and predict potential patient complications [24]. Frizzell et al. [25] used multiple ML techniques, including decision trees, gradient boosting machines, and neural networks, to predict 30-day readmissions in heart failure patients. Bayati et al. [26] applied a decision tree algorithm to determine the significant factors contributing to heart failure readmissions. Shams et al. [27] compared logistic regression, decision trees, and neural networks for their efficiency in predicting readmissions for specific diseases. Cheng et al. [28] focused on ICU transfers, which can relate to readmission rates, employing various ML models, including logistic regression and support vector machines, to predict patient deterioration. Nguyen et al. [29]

utilized logistic regression to use EHR data from entire hospital stays to predict readmissions, emphasizing the richness of hospital data in predictive modeling.

3.2 Unsupervised Learning in Healthcare Analytics

Unsupervised learning, a branch of ML, involves modeling with datasets that don't have labeled responses [30]. The system tries to learn the patterns and the structure from the input data without any labeled outcomes to guide the learning process. In healthcare, unsupervised learning has shown significant promise in patient segmentation, categorizing patients into distinct groups based on similarities in their data, which can help deliver more personalized and effective healthcare services. Unsupervised learning helps classify patients into different risk categories, enabling healthcare providers to tailor interventions and allocate resources effectively [31]. By identifying subgroups of patients with similar characteristics or conditions, healthcare providers can offer more personalized and targeted care. Identifying patient segments allows healthcare institutions to optimize resource allocation and improve service delivery. EHRs and other clinical data are used to identify patterns and segment patients based on their medical histories and health status [32]. Incorporating lifestyle and behavioral data can lead to more comprehensive patient segments and better insights into patient needs. The success of unsupervised learning depends on the quality of the data and adequate preprocessing to handle missing or noisy data. The results of unsupervised learning can be challenging to interpret and validate, necessitating a careful approach to model selection and evaluation.

In healthcare analytics, unsupervised learning can be instrumental in clustering, dimensionality reduction, and anomaly detection, among other applications. Huang et al. [33] employed SVM which is often seen in supervised settings, in an unsupervised manner for tasks like clustering. This study applied SVM in an unsupervised way for cancer genomics. Cheng et al. [34] used deep autoencoders, an unsupervised neural network, for dimensionality reduction and representation learning from EHRs. Miotto et al. [35] used deep learning (specifically, deep autoencoders) in an unsupervised manner to derive patient representations from EHR data, facilitating various predictive tasks. Buczak and Guven [36] reviewed the application of unsupervised methods, including clustering, to detect intrusions. Although this study is centered on cybersecurity, the healthcare sector is increasingly concerned with securing its data. Tian et al. [37] leveraged unsupervised ML for the identification of chronic pain patients in primary care. These studies showcase the potential of unsupervised learning in healthcare analytics, from genomics to patient record analysis.

3.3 Deep Learning Techniques in Healthcare Analytics

Deep learning has made remarkable strides in medical imaging and genomic sequencing [38]. Utilizing neural networks with numerous layers has proven to be pivotal in analyzing vast and complex datasets, contributing significantly to advancements in healthcare. This report delves into the applications, challenges, and prospects of deep learning in medical imaging and genomic sequencing. Deep learning models have demonstrated unparalleled accuracy in interpreting medical images such as X-rays, MRIs, CT scans, and ultrasounds [39]. They aid radiologists and clinicians in the early and precise diagnosis of diseases, including cancer, neurological disorders, and cardiovascular diseases, thereby improving patient outcomes. Deep learning proficiency in identifying subtle anomalies and abnormalities in medical images ensures that deviations from normal anatomy or the presence of pathologies are promptly detected, enabling timely interventions and treatments. By automating the analysis of medical images, deep learning reduces the workload on healthcare professionals, speeds up diagnosis, decreases human error, and enhances the overall efficiency of healthcare delivery.

Deep learning algorithms scrutinize genomic sequences to identify gene variants, mutations, and alterations. This analysis is crucial for understanding the genetic basis of disorders, unveiling the complexities of genetic diseases, and contributing to the development of personalized medicine. Analyzing genomic data with deep learning allows for predictions regarding individual susceptibility to various conditions. This predictive capability is instrumental in formulating preventive strategies, tailoring treatments, and understanding the hereditary nature of diseases. Deep learning accelerates drug discovery by sifting through vast genomic datasets to identify potential drug targets and predict drug responses, thereby reducing the time and cost of bringing new drugs to market.

The success of deep learning hinges on the availability and quality of large datasets. Acquiring such datasets, particularly in healthcare, is challenging due to privacy concerns, data heterogeneity, and issues related to data annotation. The complex nature of deep learning models often leads to a lack of interpretability, making it challenging for clinicians to understand and trust the model's predictions and decisions, which is vital for widespread clinical adoption. The computational demands of deep learning models are substantial. The need for powerful hardware, efficient algorithms, and considerable energy consumption can be limiting factors, especially in resource-constrained settings. Ongoing research and development are expected to yield more sophisticated and efficient deep learning algorithms. These advancements will enhance the accuracy and applicability of deep learning in medical imaging and genomic sequencing. Integrating medical imaging and genomic data through deep learning models promises to provide more comprehensive and holistic insights into patient health, leading to better diagnosis and personalized treatment strategies.

Deep learning has emerged as a transformative force in healthcare, particularly in medical imaging and genomic sequencing. Its applications extend from enhancing diagnostic precision and anomaly detection to unraveling the intricacies of the human genome and accelerating drug discovery. While challenges such as data availability, model interpretability, and computational requirements persist, the future of deep learning in these fields is promising. Continued advancements in algorithms, integrative analysis, and ethical and regulatory developments are anticipated to propel the integration of deep learning into healthcare, heralding a new era of medical innovation and personalized medicine.

Deep learning has seen significant growth in healthcare analytics due to its ability to handle vast amounts of data and derive intricate patterns. Shickel et al. [10]'s thorough survey that explores various deep learning models like Convolutional Neural Networks (CNNs) and Recurrent Neural Networks (RNNs) applied to EHR data. Rajkomar et al. [40] shed light on the broader application of ML, including deep learning in medicine, discussing challenges and opportunities. Ghassemi et al. [41] provide a deep dive into the real-world challenges and best practices for implementing AI, especially deep learning, in healthcare datasets. Esteva et al. [42] offer an overview of deep learning applications in various healthcare areas, emphasizing the transformative potential and current challenges. Gulshan et al. [43] developed a deep learning algorithm for detecting diabetic retinopathy, a cause of blindness, from eye images.

3.4 Reinforcement Learning Techniques in Healthcare Analytics

Reinforcement Learning (RL), a subset of ML, refers to the training of models to make sequences of decisions by rewarding or penalizing actions to maximize some notion of cumulative reward. In healthcare, this technique is increasingly leveraged to optimize treatment strategies, enabling personalized and adaptive medical interventions. This report explores the applications, challenges, and prospects of reinforcement learning in treatment optimization. Reinforcement learning models assist in tailoring medical interventions based on individual patient characteristics, clinical history, and real-time health data, thus contributing to more effective and personalized treatment strategies. RL algorithms adapt treatment regimens dynamically by learning from the ongoing patient responses and adjusting dosage, timing, and type of intervention to optimize therapeutic outcomes. RL-based systems serve as a decision support tool for clinicians, suggesting optimal treatment strategies, considering both short-term and long-term outcomes, and incorporating the latest clinical guidelines and research.

The inherent ability of RL to continuously learn and adapt to new data allows for dynamic adjustments to treatment plans as patients' conditions evolve, enhancing the overall efficacy of interventions. RL can optimize treatment strategies even with limited patient data by exploring different treatment options and learning from the outcomes, thus being particularly valuable in scenarios with sparse data. RL focuses on maximizing cumulative rewards, making it suitable for healthcare applications where the goal is to optimize long-term health outcomes rather than short-term gains. RL holds significant promise in optimizing treatment strategies in healthcare through its ability to personalize medicine, adapt treatment regimens, and support clinical decision-making. While safety concerns, data privacy, and model interpretability need addressing, advancements in technology and research are likely to mitigate these issues and expand the implementation of RL in treatment optimization. The integration of RL with other learning approaches and developments in safe exploration techniques further underpins its potential to revolutionize healthcare by contributing to more effective and patient-centric treatment strategies.

RL in healthcare can be particularly useful in modeling sequential decision-making problems, like treatment planning. Nemati et al. [44] use RL to determine optimal medication dosing strategies using clinical examples. Komorowski et al. [45] leveraged deep RL techniques to develop treatment strategies for sepsis treatment based on patient data. Yu et al. [46] provide a comprehensive survey on the applications and challenges of RL in various healthcare domains, providing a broad perspective on its potential and limitations.

4. IoT in Healthcare

The IoT is a transformative force in healthcare, fostering a connected environment where many devices and systems interact, share data, and contribute to improved health outcomes. By embedding technology into healthcare delivery, IoT enhances accessibility, efficiency, and patient-centric care. This report provides an in-depth exploration of the basics of IoT, its applications in patient monitoring and hospital infrastructure, and the imperative of ensuring data security and privacy. IoT in healthcare encompasses a variety of sensors, devices, and connectivity options, each serving a specific purpose in collecting, transmitting, and analyzing health-related data. Sensors are the fundamental components responsible for managing various types of health data, including vital signs, environmental conditions, and patient activity. Medical devices with sensors, such as glucose monitors, smart inhalers, and ECG monitors, capture real-time health information and transmit it for further analysis or immediate action.

Remote Patient Monitoring (RPM) and wearables represent significant applications of IoT in healthcare. RPM enables healthcare providers to remotely monitor patients' health data, aiding in chronic disease management, post-operative care, and preventive interventions. It reduces hospitalization rates and healthcare costs while improving patient' quality of life. Wearable devices like smartwatches, fitness trackers, and heart rate monitors allow individuals to monitor their health and wellness. These devices encourage proactive health management and facilitate timely medical interventions. IoT is instrumental in optimizing hospital and clinical infrastructure, enhancing patient care and operational efficiency. Smart beds, equipped with sensors, can detect patient movements, occupancy, and vital signs, ensuring optimal comfort and safety. They also alert healthcare staff to potential issues, such as patient falls or distress. IoT-based asset tracking solutions enable hospitals to monitor the location and status of medical equipment in real time. This minimizes equipment loss, optimizes asset utilization, and reduces delays in patient care.

4.1 Problems Associated with Integration of IoT and ML with Healthcare Analytics

While ML and IoT can provide transformative benefits to healthcare, the seamless integration of these technologies remains a challenge. The integration challenge, particularly in the convergence of ML and the IoT in healthcare, encompasses a broad spectrum of issues. This includes integration of diverse data streams, real-time analytics, and varying device standards. With an array of IoT devices collecting various types of data in healthcare (e.g., wearables, bedside monitors, smart equipment), assimilating them into cohesive and actionable insights is non-trivial. Kaur and Kushwaha [47] discussed the challenges of integrating vast amounts of data from IoT devices and presents methodologies and technologies to tackle this problem. Processing and acting on data in real-time, especially for critical scenarios like patient monitoring or emergency response, is both essential and challenging. Masengo Wa Umba et al. [48] describe the necessity of real-time analytics in AI-driven systems, discussing potential architectures and algorithmic solutions, which can be relevant to healthcare applications. IoT devices come from various manufacturers and can adhere to different standards. Ensuring they can communicate seamlessly and that data can be interpreted consistently is a significant hurdle. Ganzha et al. [49] provide an in-depth look into the interoperability challenges in IoT, discussing various strategies and techniques to achieve seamless device communication and integration. Rana et al. [50] delve deep into the interoperability issues faced by IoT systems, offering potential solutions and approaches to integrate devices with diverse standards.

The integration of ML and IoT in healthcare analytics has also raised concerns over data security and privacy. As endpoints they often communicate with centralized servers or other devices, IoT devices can be vulnerable to cyberattacks, potentially compromising patient data. Alaba et al. [51] provide a comprehensive survey on IoT security, including potential vulnerabilities and the current techniques used to secure IoT devices. With healthcare data being used to train and validate ML models, there are concerns that patient-specific information might be reverse-engineered from these models. Fredrikson et al. [52] highlighted how attackers can exploit ML models to extract private information, emphasizing the importance of adopting privacy-preserving ML techniques. As the number of connected devices grows and data is shared across networks, there's an increasing risk of data breaches or unauthorized data access. Mohsin et al. [53] elaborate the data-centric vulnerabilities in IoT networks, emphasizing the need for strong encryption and advanced security measures. Concerns about who owns patient data and how it's shared among healthcare providers, researchers, and third parties are paramount. Dai et al. [54] presented the potential of blockchain technology in ensuring transparent and secure data ownership and sharing in IoT networks, which is particularly relevant for sensitive healthcare data. Healthcare data is subjected to various regional and global regulations, ensuring data privacy and security, which organizations need to be aware of and comply with. Mustafa et al. [55] offered an analysis of the GDPR requirements related to healthcare data processing, emphasizing the importance of regulatory compliance for ensuring patient data privacy and security.

ML models, especially DL models, are often seen as "black boxes". In a field as critical as healthcare, this raises concerns because healthcare professionals and patients alike want to understand decisions made by the algorithms. The transparency and interpretability of ML models, particularly deep learning, are essential in domains like healthcare where decisions have critical, sometimes life-altering implications. Understanding these models ensures that medical professionals can trust and correctly act on the insights they provide. For medical professionals to trust and act upon ML predictions, they need to comprehend how decisions are made, ensuring that the model's logic aligns with medical knowledge and intuition. Holzinger et al. [56] discuss the need for and challenges of building explainable AI systems specifically tailored for the medical domain. Ribeiro et al. [57] introduced Anchors, a model-agnostic method that offers high-precision explanations, which can be valuable for understanding intricate models in healthcare settings.

DL models, especially with their deep architectures and non-linearities, are inherently more challenging to interpret than simpler models. Samek et al. [58] explore this issue making deep learning models interpretable, offering techniques and perspectives on achieving explainable AI in contexts like healthcare. While simpler models may be more interpretable, they might not always offer the best performance and balancing these considerations is vital in healthcare. Rudin [59] discusses the trade-off between model complexity and interpretability, advocating for the use of interpretable models, especially in high-stakes situations like healthcare. Visualization tools can make even complex models more comprehensible by graphically representing the model's decision-making logic. Hohman et al. [60] emphasize the role of visual analytics in demystifying deep learning models, presenting potential techniques and methods to make models more interpretable through visualization.

Data bias, fairness, and ethical considerations are paramount, especially in the healthcare domain. Hence, the reliance on historical data can inadvertently perpetuate systemic biases, making it critical to address these issues proactively. ML models trained on biased data can produce biased outcomes. In healthcare, this might mean some groups receive lower-quality care based on model recommendations. Rajkomar et al. [40] highlighted the challenge of bias in ML applications in healthcare and advocates for careful considerations to ensure fairness in ML-driven clinical tools. Relying heavily on automated ML-driven systems might reduce the human touch in healthcare, raising ethical questions about the role of machines in care provision. Char et al. [61] discussed the ethical dilemmas of integrating ML into healthcare, suggesting the need for robust guidelines and transparency to ensure the responsible use of technology. Sharing patient data for ML model training needs to be done with explicit patient consent and should ensure patient anonymity. Vayena et al. [62] elaborated on ethical concerns, emphasizing the importance of informed consent and responsible data-sharing practices in the realm of ML in medicine.

Researchers have been working on techniques to reduce and mitigate biases in ML models to ensure fairness in predictions. Corbett-Davies and Goel [63] offered a critical review of fairness in ML, suggesting methodologies and metrics to measure and ensure model fairness. The introduction of ML and automation might influence the job market in healthcare, which further introduces ethical and socio-economic considerations. Davenport and Kalakota [64] presented the transformative role of AI in healthcare, discussing not only its immense potential but also the socio-economic implications and challenges it might introduce. If the data used to train ML models isn't representative of the entire patient population, the model's predictions might not generalize well to all groups, leading to unequal care. Obermeyer et al. [65] examined racial bias in a widely used healthcare algorithm, emphasizing the need for careful evaluation and validation to ensure that ML models are equitable and beneficial for all patient groups.

The introduction of sophisticated technologies like ML and IoT in healthcare can inadvertently exacerbate health disparities if not addressed proactively. It's essential to consider the implications for global health and to ensure that advances are shared equitably. The latest technologies might be available in high-income countries while low- and middle-income countries lag. This disparity can lead to a widening gap in healthcare quality. Wirtz et al. [66] elaborated on the broader issue of access to essential medicines and technologies in global health, emphasizing the disparities between high-income and lower-income settings. Deploying advanced technologies might lead to increased healthcare costs, potentially making care less affordable in lower-resource settings. Sachs et al. [67] discussed the various transformations required to achieve sustainable development goals, including equitable healthcare, highlighting the economic challenges faced by low-income regions. In some cases, low-resource settings can leapfrog more traditional stages of healthcare infrastructure development through the adoption of digital health solutions. Labrique et al. [68] emphasized the potential of digital health solutions to transform healthcare delivery in low-resource settings, presenting a more optimistic view on technology's role in mitigating health disparities.

To ensure equitable deployment, there's a need for training and capacity-building initiatives in lower-resource settings to familiarize healthcare professionals with these advanced tools. Mosa et al. [69] emphasized the potential of smartphone applications in healthcare, especially in resource-constrained environments, and the necessity of adequate training and familiarization initiatives. Collaboration between governments, NGOs, and private companies can be instrumental in making advanced healthcare technologies accessible in low-resource settings. Rao et al. [70] explained how BRICS countries (Brazil, Russia, India, China, South Africa) are progressing towards universal health coverage, highlighting the role of collaborations and partnerships in this journey.

4.2 Recommended Solutions for Integration of IoT and ML with Healthcare Analytics

There is a definite need to encourage the adoption of standardized frameworks for integrating IoT and ML, ensuring smoother data flow and interoperability. This can be achieved to some extent through collaboration between tech developers, clinicians, and healthcare administrators. With varied devices and systems in the healthcare domain, there's a need for standardized data protocols to ensure that all systems can communicate effectively and seamlessly. Li et al. [71] presented a comprehensive framework for IoT-enabled healthcare, emphasizing the importance of standardized data protocols for efficient system communication. Collaborative efforts between tech developers, clinicians, and administrators can foster the development of standardized tools and platforms tailored for healthcare. Ting et al. [72] emphasize the necessity of collaboration between different stakeholders in harnessing technology for healthcare. Promoting open-source platforms can enable a wider community to contribute to the development of standardized frameworks and tools. Esteva et al. [42] emphasize the role of open-source initiatives in accelerating the development and adoption of ML tools in medicine. Training programs that bridge the gap between medical professionals and technologists can facilitate the creation and adoption of standardized frameworks. Topol [73] highlighted the convergence of human intelligence and artificial intelligence in medicine and underscores the importance of interdisciplinary training to harness this potential effectively. Regulatory bodies can play a pivotal role in setting and promoting standards for the integration of IoT and ML in healthcare. Char et al. [61] explored the challenges posed by AI in healthcare, including the need for regulatory standards to ensure ethical and effective deployment of technology.

The security of healthcare data, especially when using IoT devices and ML, is of paramount importance. Enhanced encryption techniques and robust security protocols are indispensable. Encryption helps ensure that the data, whether stored (at rest) or being transferred (in transit), remains confidential and only accessible to authorized entities. Bansod et al. [74] discussed the development of encryption techniques specifically tailored for IoT devices, considering their resource constraints. Xu et al. [75] highlighted the challenges of maintaining information security in the era of big data, proposing solutions for privacy and data mining, especially pertinent to healthcare.

IoT devices in healthcare, such as wearable monitors, need secure connections to avoid unauthorized access or data breaches. Alaba et al. [51] conducted a comprehensive survey covering various aspects of IoT security, emphasizing the need for secure connectivity, especially in sensitive sectors like healthcare. With evolving cyber threats, it's crucial for healthcare organizations to conduct periodic security audits and apply necessary patches or updates. Roman et al. [76] analyzed the security threats in the realm of mobile edge computing and the IoT, emphasizing the importance of regular audits and updates. Blockchain technology offers a decentralized way of maintaining data integrity and security, making it an interesting solution for healthcare applications. Liang et al. [77] discussed the potential benefits of integrating blockchain technology in mobile healthcare applications, underscoring its role in ensuring data security and facilitating collaboration

Model interpretability and explain ability are vital, especially in critical areas like healthcare where decisions can have profound implications on patient lives. Some models by design are more interpretable, such as linear regression, logistic regression, and decision trees. Rudin [59] emphasized the significance of using interpretable models, especially in high-stakes decisions such as those in healthcare. Molnar [78] offered a deep dive into various methods, including SHAP and LIME, to make ML models more explainable. Visualization tools can help in understanding the decision-making process of models, enhancing their trustworthiness. Visualization techniques were employed to make the decision-making of deep learning models more transparent in identifying metastatic breast cancer [79].

Offering training programs and workshops to healthcare professionals can help demystify ML models and build trust in their predictions. Topol [73] discussed the synergy of human intelligence and AI in medicine, highlighting the importance of educating healthcare professionals about AI and ML. Combining simple interpretable models with complex models can sometimes offer a good balance between performance and interpretability. Zhou [80] explain hybrid models and weakly supervised learning, suggesting ways to integrate simplicity and complexity for effective, yet interpretable, ML models in healthcare.

Bias mitigation and equitable access to advanced technologies are essential considerations for any responsible deployment of ML and IoT in healthcare. ML models can inherit biases present in the training data. Detecting and correcting these biases can ensure that models make fair predictions. Obermeyer et al. [65] highlight the racial bias present in an algorithm widely used in the U.S. healthcare system and underscores the importance of identifying and correcting such biases. Regular audits and evaluations of models, especially when introduced to new data sets, can ensure they remain unbiased over time. Suresh and Guttag [81] provide a framework to understand and mitigate unintended consequences, including biases in ML. Training models on diverse data sets can make them more generalizable and reduce the chances of biases related to race, gender, or other demographics. Chen et al. [82] discuss the potential of AI to either exacerbate or alleviate health disparities, highlighting the importance of diverse and representative data. Forming collaborations between high-tech regions and less resourced areas can facilitate the transfer of technology and knowledge. Spreadbury et al. [83] explain how digital health innovations, including ML and IoT, can be harnessed for neurology, with a focus on collaboration to ensure wider access.

5. Future Research Directions

Integrating diverse data streams in real-time will become increasingly critical as IoT devices increase in healthcare, from wearable sensors to smart hospital rooms [84, 85]. Hence, future studies can focus on creating robust frameworks for data integration and real-time analytics. Personalizing healthcare interventions using data from IoT devices is an exciting direction, with the need for researchers targeting the creation of patient-specific ML models that utilize continuous data streams to optimize interventions. As the integration of ML and IoT continues to grow in healthcare, so do concerns about data security and patient privacy. Researchers need to explore advanced encryption techniques, differential privacy, and secure data-sharing protocols. Future studies should explore ensuring that ML and IoT solutions are interoperable across different healthcare systems and platforms, fostering seamless healthcare experiences [87-89]. With the vast amounts of data generated by IoT devices, moving computation closer to the data source (edge computing) can be beneficial. Research can explore edge-based ML models for faster and more efficient data processing. There is also a need to ensure that ML models are robust, especially in dynamic healthcare environments where IoT data can be noisy and incomplete. Future research can explore techniques to improve model robustness and reliability in these settings. As ML and IoT continue to permeate healthcare, there will be ethical implications, from data bias to consent. Hence, there is a need for a deep dive into the ethical aspects and creation of guidelines for ML and IoT applications in healthcare Roy, S. S., Krishna, P. V. and Yenduri, S [90-92].

The issue of power constraints on many IoT devices is quite relevant, and there is a need for efficient ML models. Considering these power constraint issues, exploring techniques like model quantization, pruning, and on-device training will be pivotal for sustainable growth. Researchers could also consider investigating how to design ML-driven IoT solutions that are user-friendly and can engage patients effectively, ensuring they benefit from the latest technological advancements. Beyond prototypes and pilot studies, future research should address challenges related to the large-scale deployment of ML and IoT solutions in diverse healthcare settings. The COVID-19 pandemic has accelerated the adoption of digital health tools. Hence, there is a need to explore the long-term implications of this shift and how ML and IoT can address future healthcare challenges promptly. There is also a need for designing systems where ML models can receive real-time feedback from IoT devices, allowing them to adapt and improve over time. This will be an exciting avenue for advancing healthcare analytics. While the integration of ML and IoT offers transformative potential for healthcare analytics, addressing these future research directions will be essential to realizing their full promise and ensuring that healthcare outcomes are improved globally.

6. Conclusion

Integrating healthcare analytics, ML, and IoT represents a significant advancement in healthcare delivery. This chapter has highlighted the potential of these combined technologies to refine patient care, streamline healthcare processes, and proactively address medical challenges. However, this integration is complex, with ethical dilemmas, security concerns, and practical obstacles. Technology, healthcare, and policy professionals need to address these challenges, ensuring that adopting new technologies upholds patient trust, data integrity, and fairness. Further, the necessity of adopting patient-focused strategies and addressing global health disparities is evident. The potential of technological advancements is limited if they do not cater to diverse healthcare needs across various populations.

In conclusion, as healthcare analytics converges with ML and IoT, careful navigation, rigorous research, and interdisciplinary collaboration are paramount. The evolving landscape of healthcare, bolstered by these technologies, offers significant potential. Still, its realization depends on thorough understanding, thoughtful implementation, and a commitment to patient-centric outcomes and global equity.

References

[1] Zaouiat, C.A. and Latif, A. Internet of things and machine learning convergence: The e-healthcare revolution. *In:* Proceedings of the 2nd International Conference on Computing and Wireless Communication Systems. 2017.

[2] Weenk, M., van Goor, H., Frietman, B., Engelen, L.J., van Laarhoven, C.J., Smit, J. et al. Continuous monitoring of vital signs using wearable devices on the general ward: pilot study. JMIR mHealth and uHealth, 5(7): e7208, 2017.

[3] Ullah, M., Hamayun, S., Wahab, A., Khan, S.U., Rehman, M.U., Haq, Z.U. et al. Smart technologies used as smart tools in the management of cardiovascular disease and their future perspective. Current Problems in Cardiology, 48(11): 101922, 2023.

[4] Javaid, M., Haleem, A., Singh, R.P., Suman, R. and Rab, S. Significance of machine learning in healthcare: Features, pillars and applications. International Journal of Intelligent Networks, 3: 58-73, 2022.

[5] Padhi, A., Agarwal, A., Saxena, S.K. and Katoch, C. Transforming clinical virology with AI, machine learning and deep learning: a comprehensive review and outlook. VirusDisease, 1-11, 2023.

[6] Zeadally, S. and Bello, O. Harnessing the power of Internet of Things based connectivity to improve healthcare. Internet of Things, 14: 100074, 2021.

[7] Guni, A., Normahani, P., Davies, A. and Jaffer, U. Harnessing machine learning to personalize web-based health care content. Journal of Medical Internet Research, 23(10): e25497, 2021.

[8] Hegde, P. and Maddikunta, P.K.R. Amalgamation of Blockchain with resource-constrained IoT devices for Healthcare applications–State of Art, Challenges and

Future Directions. International Journal of Cognitive Computing in Engineering, 2023.

[9] Malik, M., Abdallah, S. and Ala'raj, M. Data mining and predictive analytics applications for the delivery of healthcare services: A systematic literature review. Annals of Operations Research, 270: 287-312, 2018.

[10] Shickel, B., Tighe, P.J., Bihorac, A. and Rashidi, P. Deep EHR: a survey of recent advances in deep learning techniques for electronic health record (EHR) analysis. IEEE Journal of Biomedical and Health *i*nformatics, 22(5): 1589-1604, 2017.

[11] Raghupathi, W. and Raghupathi, V. Big data analytics in healthcare: Promise and potential. Health Information Science and Systems, 2: 1-10, 2014.

[12] Deka, G.C. Big data predictive and prescriptive analytics. *In:* Handbook of Research on Cloud Infrastructures for Big Data Analytics. IGI Global, 370-391, 2014.

[13] Lemon, S.C., Roy, J., Clark, M.A., Friedmann, P.D. and Rakowski, W. Classification and regression tree analysis in public health: methodological review and comparison with logistic regression. Annals of Behavioral Medicine, 26: 172-181, 2003.

[14] Sukumar, S.R. and Ferrell, R.K. 'Big Data'collaboration: Exploring, recording and sharing enterprise knowledge. Information Services & Use, 33(3-4): 257-270, 2013.

[15] Božić, V. Transforming healthcare with artifical intelligence: The role of artificial intelligence in smart hospitals. Transforming Healthcare with Big Data and AI, 43(1): 145-162, 2020.

[16] Ranschaert, E., Topff, L. and Pianykh, O. Optimization of radiology workflow with artificial intelligence. Radiologic Clinics, 59(6): 955-966, 2021.

[17] Langlotz, C.P., Allen, B., Erickson, B.J., Kalpathy-Cramer, J., Bigelow, K., Cook, T.S. et al. A roadmap for foundational research on artificial intelligence in medical imaging: From the 2018 NIH/RSNA/ACR/The Academy Workshop. Radiology, 291(3): 781-791, 2019.

[18] Mbunge, E., Muchemwa, B. and Batani, J. Sensors and healthcare 5.0: Transformative shift in virtual care through emerging digital health technologies. Global Health Journal, 5(4): 169-177, 2021.

[19] Alfian, G., Syafrudin, M., Ijaz, M.F., Syaekhoni, M.A., Fitriyani, N.L. and Rhee, J. A personalized healthcare monitoring system for diabetic patients by utilizing BLE-based sensors and real-time data processing. Sensors, 18(7): 2183, 2018.

[20] Shouval, R., Bondi, O., Mishan, H., Shimoni, A., Unger, R. and Nagler, A. Application of machine learning algorithms for clinical predictive modeling: a data-mining approach in SCT. Bone Marrow Transplantation, 49(3): 332-337, 2014.

[21] Yun, C., Shun, M., Junta, U. and Browndi, I. Predictive analytics: A survey, trends, applications, opportunities' and challenges for smart city planning. International Journal of Computer Science and Information Technology, 23(56): 226-231, 2022.

[22] Goodney, P.P., Stukel, T.A., Lucas, F.L., Finlayson, E.V. and Birkmeyer, J.D. Hospital volume, length of stay, and readmission rates in high-risk surgery. Annals of Surgery, 238(2): 161, 2003.

[23] Caruana, R., Lou, Y., Gehrke, J., Koch, P., Sturm, M. and Elhadad, N. Intelligible models for healthcare: Predicting pneumonia risk and hospital 30-day readmission. *In:* Proceedings of the 21th ACM SIGKDD International Conference on Knowledge Discovery and Data Mining. 2015.

[24] Cox, J.C., Sadiraj, V., Schnier, K.E. and Sweeney, J.F. Incentivizing cost-effective reductions in hospital readmission rates. Journal of Economic Behavior & Organization, 131: 24-35, 2016.

[25] Frizzell, J.D., Liang, L., Schulte, P.J., Yancy, C.W., Heidenreich, P.A., Hernandez, A.F. et al. Prediction of 30-day all-cause readmissions in patients hospitalized for heart failure: Comparison of machine learning and other statistical approaches. JAMA Cardiology, 2(2): 204-209, 2017.
[26] Bayati, M., Braverman, M., Gillam, M., Mack, K.M., Ruiz, G., Smith, M.S. and Horvitz, E. Data-driven decisions for reducing readmissions for heart failure: General methodology and case study. PloS One, 9(10): e109264, 2014.
[27] Shams, I., Ajorlou, S. and Yang, K. A predictive analytics approach to reducing 30-day avoidable readmissions among patients with heart failure, acute myocardial infarction, pneumonia, or COPD. Health Care Management Science, 18: 19-34, 2015.
[28] Cheng, F.-Y., Joshi, H., Tandon, P., Freeman, R., Reich, D.L., Mazumdar, M. et al. Using machine learning to predict ICU transfer in hospitalized COVID-19 patients. Journal of Clinical Medicine, 9(6): 1668, 2020.
[29] Nguyen, O.K., Makam, A.N., Clark, C., Zhang, S., Xie, B., Velasco, F., Amarasingham, R. and Halm, E.A. Predicting all-cause readmissions using electronic health record data from the entire hospitalization: Model development and comparison. Journal of Hospital Medicine, 11(7): 473-480, 2016.
[30] Hiran, K.K., Jain, R.K., Lakhwani, K. and Doshi, R. Machine Learning: Master Supervised and Unsupervised Learning Algorithms with Real Examples (English Edition). BPB Publications, 2021.
[31] Dogheim, G.M. and Hussain, A. Patient care through AI-driven remote monitoring: Analyzing the role of predictive models and intelligent alerts in preventive medicine. Journal of Contemporary Healthcare Analytics, 7(1): 94-110, 2023.
[32] Thyvalikakath, T.P., Dziabiak, M.P., Johnson, R., Torres-Urquidy, M.H., Acharya, A., Yabes, J. and Schleyer, T.K. Advancing cognitive engineering methods to support user interface design for electronic health records. International Journal of Medical Informatics, 83(4): 292-302, 2014.
[33] Huang, S., Cai, N., Pacheco, P.P., Narrandes, S., Wang, Y. and Xu, W. Applications of support vector machine (SVM) learning in cancer genomics. Cancer Genomics & Proteomics, 15(1): 41-51, 2018.
[34] Cheng, Y., Wang, F., Zhang, P. and Hu, J. Risk prediction with electronic health records: A deep learning approach. *In:* Proceedings of the 2016 SIAM International Conference in Data Mining. 2016. SIAM.
[35] Miotto, R., Li, L., Kidd, B.A. and Dudley, J.T. Deep patient: An unsupervised representation to predict the future of patients from the electronic health records. Scientific Reports, 6(1): 1-10, 2016.
[36] Buczak, A.L. and Guven, E. A survey of data mining and machine learning methods for cyber security intrusion detection. IEEE Communications Surveys & Tutorials, 18(2): 1153-1176, 2015.
[37] Tian, T.Y., Zlateva, I. and Anderson, D.R. Using electronic health records data to identify patients with chronic pain in a primary care setting. Journal of the American Medical Informatics Association, 20(e2): e275-e280, 2013.
[38] Lee, J.-G., Jun, S., Cho, Y.-W., Lee, H., Kim, G.B., Seo, J.B. and Kim, N. Deep learning in medical imaging: General overview. Korean Journal of Radiology, 18(4): 570-584, 2017.
[39] Wang, J., Zhu, H., Wang, S.-H. and Zhang, Y.-D. A review of deep learning on medical image analysis. Mobile Networks and Applications, 26: 351-380, 2021.
[40] Rajkomar, A., Dean, J. and Kohane, I. Machine learning in medicine. New England Journal of Medicine, 380(14): 1347-1358, 2019.

[41] Ghassemi, M., Naumann, T., Schulam, P., Beam, A.L., Chen, I.Y. and Ranganath, R. Practical guidance on artificial intelligence for health-care data. The Lancet Digital Health, 1(4): e157-e159, 2019.

[42] Esteva, A., Robicquet, A., Ramsundar, B., Kuleshov, V., DePristo, M., Chou, K. et al. A guide to deep learning in healthcare. Nature Medicine, 25(1): 24-29, 2019.

[43] Gulshan, V., Peng, L., Coram, M., Stumpe, M.C., Wu, D., Narayanaswamy, A. et al. Development and validation of a deep learning algorithm for detection of diabetic retinopathy in retinal fundus photographs. Jama, 316(22): 2402-2410, 2016.

[44] Nemati, S., Ghassemi, M.M. and Clifford, G.D. Optimal medication dosing from suboptimal clinical examples: A deep reinforcement learning approach. *In:* 2016 38th Annual International Conference of the IEEE Engineering in Medicine and Biology Society (EMBC). 2016. IEEE.

[45] Komorowski, M., Celi, L.A., Badawi, O., Gordon, A.C. and Faisal, A.A. The artificial intelligence clinician learns optimal treatment strategies for sepsis in intensive care. Nature Medicine, 24(11): 1716-1720, 2018.

[46] Yu, C., Liu, J., Nemati, S. and Yin, G. Reinforcement learning in healthcare: A survey. ACM Computing Surveys (CSUR), 55(1): 1-36, 2021.

[47] Kaur, H. and Kushwaha, A.S. A review on integration of big data and IoT. *In:* 2018 4th International Conference on Computing Sciences (ICCS). 2018. IEEE.

[48] Masengo Wa Umba, S., Abu-Mahfouz, A.M. and Ramotsoela, D. Artificial intelligence-driven intrusion detection in software-defined wireless sensor networks: Towards secure IoT-enabled healthcare systems. International Journal of Environmental Research and Public Health, 19(9): 5367, 2022.

[49] Ganzha, M., Paprzycki, M., Pawłowski, W., Szmeja, P. and Wasielewska, K. Semantic interoperability in the Internet of Things: An overview from the INTER-IoT perspective. Journal of Network and Computer Applications, 81: 111-124, 2017.

[50] Rana, B., Singh, Y. and Singh, P.K. A systematic survey on internet of things: Energy efficiency and interoperability perspective. Transactions on Emerging Telecommunications Technologies, 32(8): e4166, 2021.

[51] Alaba, F.A., Othman, M., Hashem, I.A.T. and Alotaibi, F. Internet of Things security: A survey. Journal of Network and Computer Applications, 88: 10-28, 2017.

[52] Fredrikson, M., Jha, S. and Ristenpart, T. Model inversion attacks that exploit confidence information and basic countermeasures. *In:* Proceedings of the 22nd ACM SIGSAC Conference on Computer And Communications Security. 2015.

[53] Mohsin, M., Anwar, Z., Zaman, F. and Al-Shaer, E. IoTChecker: A data-driven framework for security analytics of Internet of Things configurations. Computers & Security, 70: 199-223, 2017.

[54] Dai, H.-N., Zheng, Z. and Zhang, Y. Blockchain for Internet of Things: A survey. IEEE Internet of Things Journal, 6(5): 8076-8094, 2019.

[55] Mustafa, U., Pflugel, E. and Philip, N. A novel privacy framework for secure m-health applications: The case of the GDPR. *In:* 2019 IEEE 12th International Conference on Global Security, Safety and Sustainability (ICGS3). 2019. IEEE.

[56] Holzinger, A., Biemann, C., Pattichis, C.S. and Kell, D.B. What do we need to build explainable AI systems for the medical domain? arXiv preprint arXiv:1712.09923, 2017.

[57] Ribeiro, M.T., Singh, S. and Guestrin, C. Anchors: High-precision model-agnostic explanations. *In:* Proceedings of the AAAI Conference on Artificial Intelligence. 2018.

[58] Samek, W., Montavon, G., Vedaldi, A., Hansen, L.K. and Müller, K.-R. Explainable AI: Interpreting, Explaining and Visualizing Deep Learning. Vol. 11700. 2019: Springer Nature.

[59] Rudin, C. Stop explaining black box machine learning models for high stakes decisions and use interpretable models instead. Nature Machine Intelligence, 1(5): 206-215, 2019.

[60] Hohman, F., Kahng, M., Pienta, R. and Chau, D.H. Visual analytics in deep learning: An interrogative survey for the next frontiers. IEEE Transactions on Visualization and Computer Graphics, 25(8): 2674-2693, 2018.

[61] Char, D.S., Shah, N.H. and Magnus, D. Implementing machine learning in health care—Addressing ethical challenges. The New England Journal of Medicine, 378(11): 981, 2018.

[62] Vayena, E., Blasimme, A. and Cohen, I.G. Machine learning in medicine: Addressing ethical challenges. PLoS Medicine, 15(11): e1002689, 2018.

[63] Corbett-Davies, S. and Goel, S. The measure and mismeasure of fairness: A critical review of fair machine learning. arXiv preprint arXiv:1808.00023, 2018.

[64] Davenport, T. and Kalakota, R. The potential for artificial intelligence in healthcare. Future Healthcare Journal, 6(2): 94, 2019.

[65] Obermeyer, Z., Powers, B., Vogeli, C. and Mullainathan, S. Dissecting racial bias in an algorithm used to manage the health of populations. Science, 366(6464): 447-453, 2019.

[66] Wirtz, V.J., Hogerzeil, H.V., Gray, A.L., Bigdeli, M., de Joncheere, C.P., Ewen, M.A. et al. Essential medicines for universal health coverage. The Lancet, 389(10067): 403-476, 2017.

[67] Sachs, J.D., Schmidt-Traub, G., Mazzucato, M., Messner, D., Nakicenovic, N. and Rockström, J. Six transformations to achieve the sustainable development goals. Nature Sustainability, 2(9): 805-814, 2019.

[68] Labrique, A., Vasudevan, L., Mehl, G., Rosskam, E. and Hyder, A.A. Digital health and health systems of the future. Global Health: Science and Practice, S1-S4, 2018.

[69] Mosa, A.S.M., Yoo, I. and Sheets, L. A systematic review of healthcare applications for smartphones. BMC Medical Informatics and Decision Making, 12(1): 1-31, 2012.

[70] Rao, K.D., Petrosyan, V., Araujo, E.C. and McIntyre, D. Progress towards universal health coverage in BRICS: Translating economic growth into better health. Bulletin of the World Health Organization, 92: 429-435, 2014.

[71] Li, J., Cai, J., Khan, F., Rehman, A.U., Balasubramaniam, V., Sun, J. and Venu, P. A secured framework for sdn-based edge computing in IOT-enabled healthcare system. IEEE Access, 8: 135479-135490, 2020.

[72] Ting, D.S.W., Carin, L., Dzau, V. and Wong, T.Y. Digital technology and COVID-19. Nature Medicine, 26(4): 459-461, 2020.

[73] Topol, E.J., High-performance medicine: The convergence of human and artificial intelligence. Nature Medicine, 25(1): 44-56, 2019.

[74] Bansod, G., Patil, A., Sutar, S. and Pisharoty, N. ANU: An ultra lightweight cipher design for security in IoT. Security and Communication Networks, 9(18): 5238-5251, 2016.

[75] Xu, L., Jiang, C., Wang, J., Yuan, J. and Ren, Y. Information security in big data: Privacy and data mining. IEEE Access, 2: 1149-1176, 2014.

[76] Roman, R., Lopez, J. and Mambo, M. Mobile edge computing, fog: A survey and analysis of security threats and challenges. Future Generation Computer Systems, 78: 680-698, 2018.

[77] Liang, X., Zhao, J., Shetty, S., Liu, J. and Li, D. Integrating blockchain for data sharing and collaboration in mobile healthcare applications. *In:* 2017 IEEE 28th Annual International Symposium on Personal, Indoor, and Mobile Radio Communications (PIMRC). 2017. IEEE.

[78] Molnar, C., Interpretable machine learning. Lulu.com, 2020.

[79] Wang, D., Khosla, A., Gargeya, R., Irshad, H. and Beck, A.H. Deep learning for identifying metastatic breast cancer. arXiv preprint arXiv:1606.05718, 2016.

[80] Zhou, Z.-H. A brief introduction to weakly supervised learning. National Science Review, 5(1): 44-53, 2018.

[81] Suresh, H. and Guttag, J.V. A framework for understanding unintended consequences of machine learning. arXiv preprint arXiv:1901.10002, 2(8), 2019.

[82] Chen, I.Y., Szolovits, P. and Ghassemi, M. Can AI help reduce disparities in general medical and mental health care? AMA Journal of Ethics, 21(2): 167-179, 2019.

[83] Spreadbury, J.H., Young, A. and Kipps, C.M. A comprehensive literature search of digital health technology use in neurological conditions: Review of digital tools to promote self-management and support. Journal of Medical Internet Research, 24(7): e31929, 2022.

[84] Kute, S., Tyagi, A.K., Sahoo, R. and Malik, S. Building a smart healthcare system using Internet of Things and machine learning. Big Data Biomedical Data Analysis: Current Status and Future Trends, 321: 159-178, 2022.

[85] Roy, S.S., Pratyush, C. and Barna, C. Predicting ozone layer concentration using multivariate adaptive regression splines, random forest and classification and regression tree. *In:* Soft Computing Applications: Proceedings of the 7th International Workshop Soft Computing Applications (SOFA 2016), 27: 140-152. 2018. Springer International Publishing.

[86] Roy, S.S., Gupta, A., Sinha, A. and Ramesh, R. Cancer data investigation using variable precision rough set with flexible classification. *In:* Proceedings of the Second International Conference on Computational Science, Engineering and Information Technology, 472-475. 2012, October.

[87] Bose, A., Roy, S.S., Balas, V.E. and Samui, P. Deep learning for brain computer interfaces. Handbook of Deep Learning Applications, 333-344, 2019.

[88] Roy, S.S. and Taguchi, Y.H. Identification of genes associated with altered gene expression and m6A profiles during hypoxia using tensor decomposition based unsupervised feature extraction. Scientific Reports, 11(1): 8909, 2021.

[89] Chakraborty, C., Bhattacharya, M., Sharma, A.R., Roy, S.S., Islam, M.A., Chakraborty, S. et al. Deep learning research should be encouraged for diagnosis and treatment of antibiotic resistance of microbial infections in treatment associated emergencies in hospitals. International Journal of Surgery, 105: 106857, 2022.

[90] Roy, S.S., Krishna, P.V. and Yenduri, S. Analyzing intrusion detection system: An ensemble-based stacking approach. *In:* 2014 IEEE International Symposium on Signal Processing and Information Technology (ISSPIT), 000307-000309, 2014, December. IEEE.

[91] Bandhu, A. and Roy, S.S. Classifying multi-category images using deep learning: A convolutional neural network model. *In:* 2017 2nd IEEE International Conference on Recent Trends in Electronics, Information & Communication Technology (RTEICT), 915-919, 2017, May. IEEE.

[92] Li, W., Chai, Y., Khan, F., Jan, S.R.U., Verma, S., Menon, V.G. et al. A comprehensive survey on machine learning-based big data analytics for IoT-enabled smart healthcare system. Mobile Networks and Applications, 26: 234-252, 2021.

CHAPTER

4

A Study Aimed at Presenting Methodologies for Enhancing Cost Efficiency in Healthcare Systems Based on Internet of Things (IoT) by Incorporating Sophisticated Deep Learning and Artificial Intelligence Techniques

Oishik Ghosh*

University of Manchester, Manchester, United Kingdom

The Internet of Things, sometimes known as IoT, is a network made up of interconnected human beings, computer-based gadgets, and occasionally inanimate home items that are in charge of exchanging data with one another. These gadgets are frequently wearable or function as a remote monitoring system. This chapter examines several strategies to reduce the time and resources required to choose the best network plan, sensor configuration, and data extraction and transformation. A comprehensive examination of case studies is subsequently performed with the intention of deducing conclusions from contemporary cost effective measures.

1. Overview of Implementation in Healthcare

In order to effectively use cost reduction techniques in Healthcare Systems that are facilitated with the help of Internet of Things (IOT) devices, it is necessary

*Corresponding author: oishikg10@gmail.com

to understand the principles behind its implementation. In the modern era of healthcare systems, these IOT devices primarily contribute to automating processes that were previously reliant on human actions, some of which were often redundant. By enabling automation of these actions, it minimizes the potential for human errors and increases operational efficiency by saving time.

One such procedure that has been prevalent is known as Non-Invasive Patient Distress Monitoring [1]. This is accomplished essentially by the collection of physiological data such as the patient's blood pressure, heart rate, body temperature, and breathing rate. Such underlying information may shine light on fundamental circumstances. A blood pressure that is lower than usual, for example, could indicate Hypo-Tension, whereas a higher rate would indicate Hyper-Tension. Similarly, if the heart rate or pulse is irregular or elevated, it could be the source of cardiovascular disorders such as heart arrhythmias. Through X-Ray or MRI scans, more intricate signs such as lumpy skin patches, irregularities in bowel or bladder habits, or tissue discoloration on the skin may be symptomatic of early cancer. With the help of smart wearable equipment and remote monitoring systems, these IOT devices are responsible for collecting physiological data.

Engel et al. [2] propose a commonly used approach for setting the IOT Interface to undergo monitoring in specific contexts. The method may be broken down into three main stages: choosing the right sensor, extracting and transforming the data, and then diagnosing the problem using deep learning algorithms and neural networks. In this chapter, we go over how to choose sensors wisely, plan a network's architecture, and extract and process data effectively. Finally, we examine case studies using current deep learning methodologies on information gathered from IoT devices and make conclusions.

2. Sensor Selection and Energy Optimization Techniques

There are two types of IOT Interface Setups that can be utilised to collect data from patients [3]. The first is a Wireless Sensor Network (WSN), which is frequently embedded in external wearable devices or implanted inside in the patient's body. Each implanted sensor functions as a node, gathering data from those specific regions and transmitting it synchronously to a centrally assigned node. This data reaches an authorised system, which is then accountable for data-driven diagnostics. Despite the fact that it is beneficial in many ways, it consumes an exorbitant amount of energy for aggregating data and routing. There are several approaches which could be used to reduce this.

In a conventional WSN, the nodes are directly connected to each other, as shown in Fig. 1. As a result, a single node is receiving and transmitting data at the same time. Hence, at that given condition or time period, the energy consumption for both activities is relatively high.

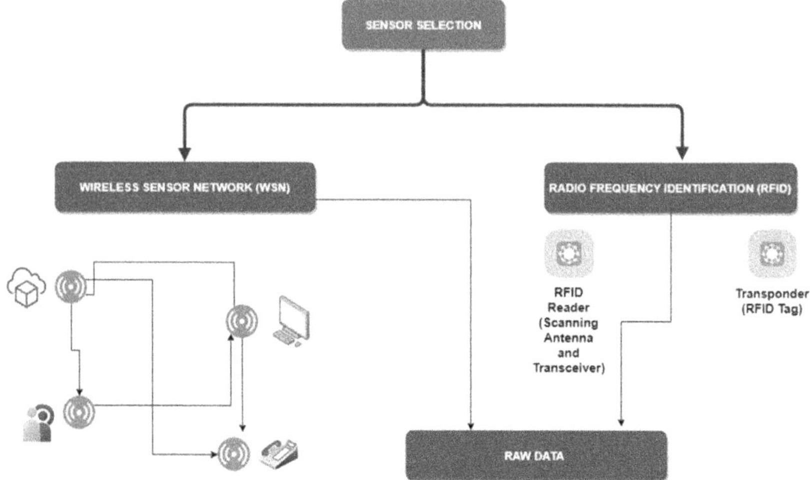

Figure 1. Sensor categorization

2.1 LEECH Protocol Techniques in WSNs

A logical approach of mitigating this would be to separate the states for the transceiver and receiver for each node [3] discuss time synchronous methods following the LEECH Protocol to resolve this issue. The main focus of the Protocol remains clustering the nodes in order to reduce the message transmission loads of a single node and applying a duty cycle. The working is shown in the diagram below.

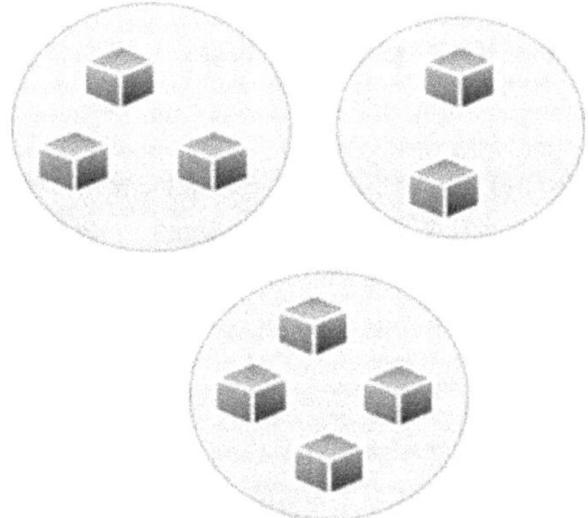

Figure 2. Clustering nodes in a WSN network

The question then becomes, what is the optimum approach to cluster the nodes? One crucial consideration in this situation is that each cluster must be mutually exclusive, as each node in Cluster C1 would thus be unable to transmit or receive data from another cluster C2. This would be a simple process if each node or sensor was only responsible for one action, such as fully studying brain responses and nothing else, or fully analysing tissue lesions and nothing else.

However, in a real-world scenario with an infinite number of sensors, it would be impossible to cluster them manually in the best feasible way. Besides, if not done correctly, it might have major repercussions, such as improper data reads causing false positives and false negatives, resulting in a critical misreading case. Hence it is necessary to use clustering algorithms. Hämäläinen, J. et al. [5] enlist several approaches to do so. Let's examine these strategies and decide which is the most effective.

The first possible approach is Euclidean distance based classical clustering such as using K Means. Since the nature of each sensor in this case is solely independent of distance, it is likely to be viewed as being less effective. The arm would have sensors for measuring the pulse, but the sensors for measuring ECG or neural signals would be spaced out at much closer intervals. Given that pure hierarchical clustering has been empirically shown to perform poorly when dealing with big data sets and mixed data types [6]; both of which are essentially guaranteed in this case, it would likewise appear unwise to utilize it.

Fuzzy logic clustering appears to be the most suited of all, because its operation involves assigning a degree of membership to each sensor node, building clusters based on the similarity of the data it collects. In accordance with the LEACH Protocol in [7] the algorithm functions in two separate states.

The first state is the set-up state, which includes numerous iterations. In each such iteration, each of the sensors is tasked with determining whether or not to act as the cluster's head. A sensor accomplishes this by obtaining a binary value of 0 or 1. There is a predetermined desired proportion P, which aids the cluster in determining it. The following formula determines the value $F(m)$ where N is the total number of iterations.

$$F(m) = \left(\frac{P}{1 - \left(P \times N \times \text{mod}\left(\frac{1}{p} \right) \right)} \right) m \epsilon G \tag{1}$$

If the selected value of the sensory node is less than $F(m)$, it remains a head in that iteration. The cluster is established by nodes that are no longer designated as heads and are sending a join-request message to their nearest head. After N iterations, the value G reflects the total number of nodes with values greater than $F(m)$. For this IoT interface to function properly, it is necessary to understand how many epochs or iterations the algorithm must go through in order to produce the most accurate results.

Since each sensory node is limited to its own cluster, the clusters formed would result in less energy consumption. However, there is still a requirement to separate the transmission phase from the receiving phase to reduce load rate (load per unit time) on an individual sensor at a certain time. This is fulfilled in the secondary state.

In the secondary steady state, a method known as Time Division Multiple Access (TDMA) is utilized to achieve that [8]. In this method, there is a predetermined bandwidth that is to be allotted to each cluster. Each sensor is allowed complete freedom to use the entire bandwidth for fast and efficient data transmission. However, the time given to each sensor is divided. So, if there are 5 sensors in the cluster namely A, B, C, D and E, the time for each round is divided into 5 parts of T_A, T_B, T_C, T_D and $T_{E.}$ Based on priority, the divisions may not necessarily be equal. The following figure illustrates the flow of time.

A total time frame is provided to each round N that remains consistent across all rounds. The purpose is that when a receiver wishes to search for transmitted information from a specific sensor, it can pre-determine the allotted slot for that sensor in a time period.

This procedure, however, has a significant limitation [9]. If a sensor does not have enough data to transmit to fully use its time slot for a particular round, it may result in left over time for that sensor's unique slot. Because the time difference between this sensor and the next is no longer consistent, the next sensor's time slot may begin improperly. As a result, to address this issue, a guard band is used between time slots to absorb the timing inconsistencies.

An effective approach for lowering the load-rate of the IOT Interface sensor has now been established. This has, however, led to the realisation that there is a cost-benefit trade-off in this case.

To better comprehend it, consider the initial time required to finish the total data transmission and receiving as T. Because of the possibility of clustering, an additional time segment ΔT_1 is used. Furthermore, the same operation takes ΔT_2 time longer in the secondary steady state due to the usage of the TDMA protocol. Thus, the new total time necessary to cut energy costs is $T+\Delta T_1+\Delta T_2$.

2.2 Energy Optimization in RFID Sensors

Radio Frequency Identification (RFID) is the secondary form of IoT Interface setup. Its operating principle differs from that of WSNs, which sense and monitor their surroundings. When it comes to continuous measurement of a physiological aspect such as heart rate, WSNs are especially prevalent for data collection [10]. However, as previously said, in order to identify the potential danger of more serious health concerns, it is occasionally necessary to detect the presence of anomalies such as lumps in the body, tissue discolouration, or platelet congestion.

A tag is attached to each patient. Each tag is in control of collecting information about the patient's body by passing radio waves. These radio waves have the capability to collect information from multiple organ areas in the human body at once, and send it to a reader. Through several such tags, information

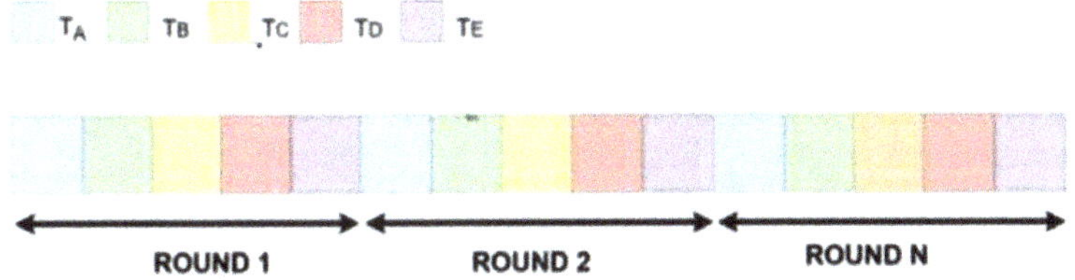

Figure 3. TDMA in the steady state

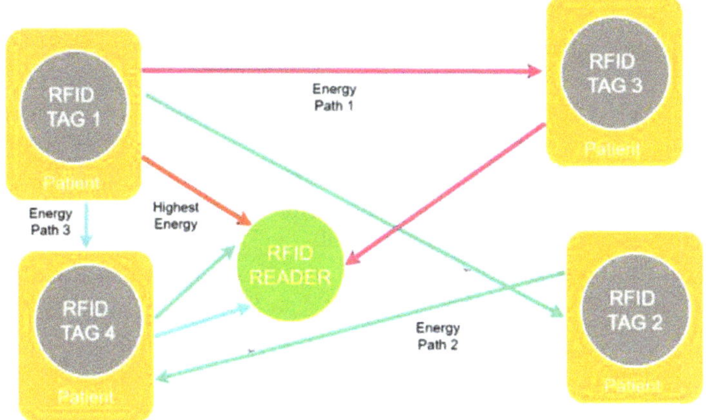

Figure 4. Potential pathways for transmitting radio waves are illustrated in this example

is gathered and stored in a database enabled with a search feature to recognize health irregularities needing a diagnosis [11].

2.2.1 Implementing Genetic Algorithm

One of the most successful methods to optimize this approach feature is using the Genetic Algorithm. The wireless network of patients with tags is quite diverse and complex in the actual world, and there is a great deal of space between them.

It can be visualised as a "tree" with each patient's tag acting as a node and the edges being identified as the path of radio waves to each node. To ensure that the minimum amount of energy is utilized to gather information, it is necessary to plan a connection path that requires minimum traversal.

Tag 1 has the possibility to transfer data to the reader directly, as seen in the example above. However, because of considerations like distance, the energy consumption in that situation is believed to be the largest. There are three additional paths that can be taken that use a lot less energy. Without having to attempt every single path combination due to time and energy constraints, the option with the lowest cost out of all of these potential solutions should be chosen.

In this algorithm, each tag can be considered as a member of an initial population. A "fitness function" is to be selected to define the fittest members in the sample population. Once selected, the fittest members can be used for cross over and mutation iteratively. Each path will be made up of a number of smaller actions, like moving north, east, west, or south. Each such action is considered as an individual "gene" while the entire path can be considered as the "DNA". Two different paths can involve common genes but the complete DNA would be unique in each case. Each gene or action at a particular time will either have a positive or negative impact on the cost needed to transmit a radio wave.

Let the initial tag take a number of possible routes to the reader at start, allotting a constant energy to each route. With that energy, some paths would have allowed radio waves to go farther than other paths. The distance covered while using a fixed amount of energy can serve as the fitness function here.

Through the process of "Selection" the top N paths are chosen based on the greatest distance travelled i.e. fitness function. The information from the paths of the fittest members is then utilized to "mutate" or combine to create a path that outperforms all other participating selected paths. To do this, each path is divided into sections, and the optimal set of actions for each sector is joined to form a combined path. This is known as "Mutation and Crossover".

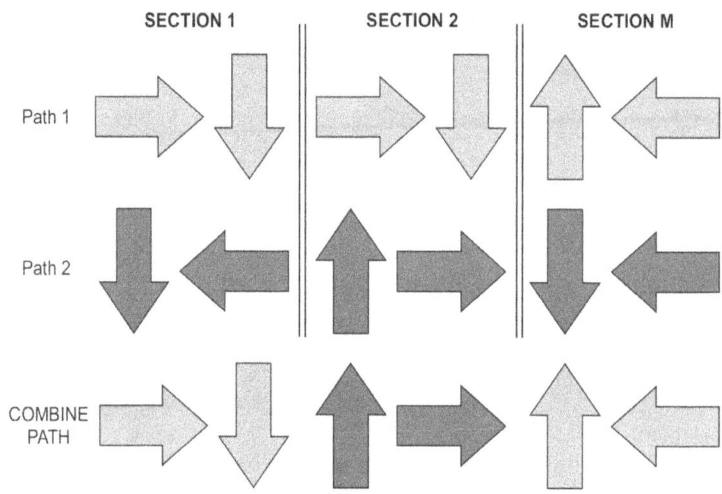

Figure 5. Illustration of mutation and crossover for the path taken by radio waves

This process is repeated over several iterations to obtain the path with the least amount of energy consumed.

2.2.2 *Probabilistic Approaches for the Mutation and Crossover Rate*

It is possible that the mutation results in reaching a Local Minima point. This might occur if a specific activity was completely overlooked for the combined path. As an illustration, the combined path only includes three of the aforementioned four acts, such as North, East, and South. If moving west is necessary, it would be impossible to do so. The memory of the unused action sequences must therefore be stored apart from the combined path.

To address this issue, a suitable "Mutation Rate" must be chosen. If the rate is set too high, the combined path may deviate from its intended endpoint (the RFID reader) after learning numerous action sequences. If it is too low, it will tend to gravitate towards the local minima. Prior studies have demonstrated that the best value is between 5% and 20%, with a small population size [13].

However, Ahmad et al. have discussed how this convention may not always provide the best results and suggested a dynamic approach known as ILM/DHC (Increasing Low Mutation/Decreasing High Crossover) to choose the mutation and crossover rates [14]. Here the Mutation Rate (MR) increases from 0 to 100% and Crossover Rate decreases from 100 to 0%. It is given by the formulation,

$$MR = \frac{G_c}{G_n}, CR = 1 - MR \tag{2}$$

Here, MR is the mutation rate while CR is the crossover rate. The current generation is denoted by G_c with G_n being the total number of generations. Even with greater population numbers, this approach has been shown to perform effectively[14]. The explanation is that the algorithm's probabilistic nature allows it to meet the need for extra crossings at higher iterations or generations. This requirement stems from the diversity in a bigger population (in our example, patients with RFID tags), which necessitates stronger crossover solutions inherited from past generations rather than mutations from the local optima.

2.2.3 *Reduction of Interference and Maximizing Coverage of a RFID Reader*

An antenna is affixed to each RFID tag. There is a significant amount of interference when trying to transmit radio waves in a large network with many tags and readers. Hence, this causes the RFID network planning (RNP) to be classified as a NP-Hard problem [15].The energy cost rises as network complexity and redundancy both increase. An effective way of reducing the interference would be to minimise the number of readers receiving the information by increasing coverage of each of them. This can be achieved by Particle Swarm Optimization (PSO).

Each particle in a "Particle Swarm" consists of a velocity vector, position vector and a previous optimal position vector. Then, based on all of these values, a team optimal location vector is determined, which is likewise communicated to each particle.

A RFID reader primarily sends power and signal instructions to the Tags, which then transmit the data back. Based on the three vectors in the example, the initial signal movement is depicted in the image on next page.

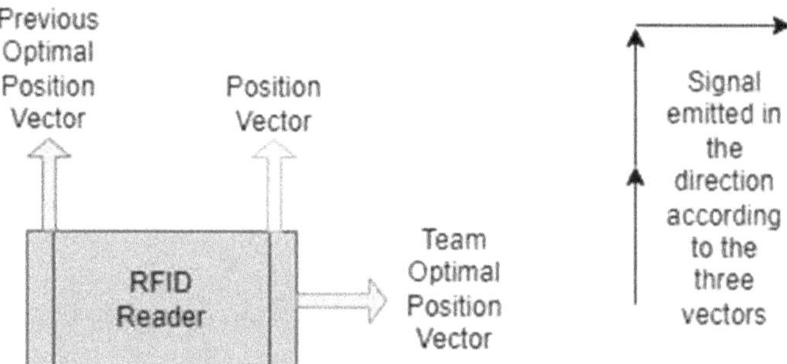

Figure 6. The route taken by a reader signals is that of PSO

If the signal reaches a position that is better than the individual or team optimal location, the value is updated at the end of the iteration. If it falls into a worse position, it only saves the present direction. Each tag eventually realises the ideal locations to transmit the information to reach the RFID reader after a specific number of iterations. It may ignore the local optima and look for a global solution.

The challenge then becomes, how do we reduce the number of readers by using this method? A reader delivers signals through the PSO route in each repetition. Following several such rounds, a coverage area for the reader can be identified, as illustrated in the image below.

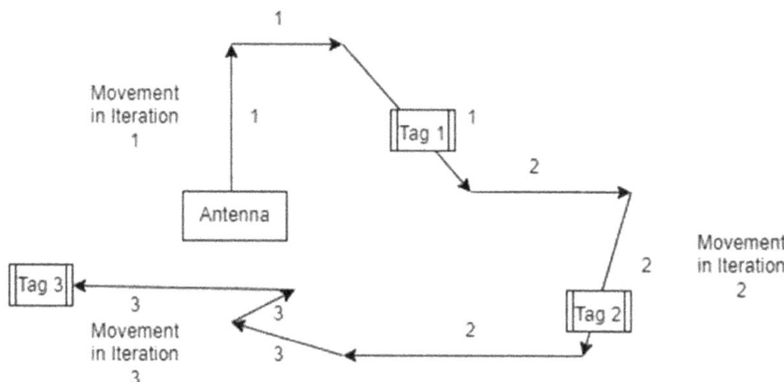

Figure 7. Coverage is contingent upon the routes of the Public Service Obligation (PSO)

In this scenario, the reader R1 takes three iterations and hence three PSO paths in order to send out signals. This path is shown to span three tags, T1, T2, and T3.

There are numerous such readers in a RNP. Assume the existence of another reader R2 who is familiar with the tags T2, T3, and T4. Let T1, T5, and T6 be the tags covered for another reader R3. The total set of tags covered by R2 and R3 in this scenario would be T1, T2, T3, T4, T5, and T6. As a result, because we can cover the first six tags with these two readers, the first reader (R1) is not required. Thus, by removing unnecessary readers, interference can be decreased using this strategy. Furthermore, as the number of iterations increases, each reader will be able to recognise more tags in its PSO path, boosting individual coverage.

By utilising these techniques, the power and energy expenses associated with the sensor selection process can be decreased. The data must first be pre-processed after it is received before being fed to a neural network or deep learning algorithm. The following section goes over this.

2.3 Raw Data Pre-processing

The Extract, Transform and Load Paradigm (ETL) is a commonly used technique to pre-process unstructured data as discussed by Shifeng Fang et al. [23]. Below, we discuss various methods for enhancing each level of the ETL, through adaptive data extraction, parallel execution of functional programming and data loading.

2.3.1 Data Extraction through an Effective Sampling Strategy

In this section, we will consider frequency-based data collecting. Data collection timeframes might differ throughout different stages of a health-based diagnosis. During COVID, for example, an Oximeter was used to measure an individual's oxygen levels. When a person is fit and healthy, it is done as a regular check-up to detect disruptions early. But when a patient is diagnosed with COVID, the oxygen levels must be tested significantly more regularly. Adaptive Sampling is a useful approach for selecting when and how frequently sensor values should be read based on dynamic requirements [16].

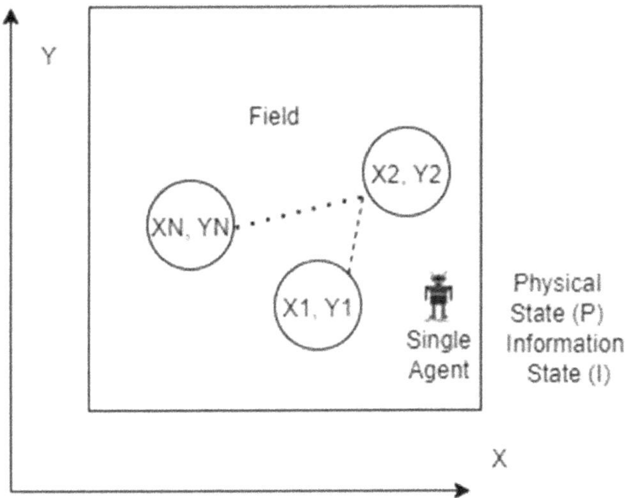

Figure 8. Sampling undertaken by single agent

There must be three considerations for this objective. First, the sensor-embedded agent has a positional realisation or physical state (P) in the spatial field. In the figure above, a single agent is initially present in a field at the coordinate (X1, Y1). Second, the sensor understands the field in which it is located. This is referred to as the Information State (I). Finally, the agent should have a "sampling strategy" that informs the robot on what course to follow or where to go next.

If the sampling approach is fixed, the agent moves in predictable patterns through the field. This happens when we already have prior knowledge of the field region. This is especially handy when a complete coverage is required rather than just locating the local maxima or minima. There is, however, a requirement of sufficient time to do so.

However, in the case of adaptive sampling, an agent samples exactly at a starting point and changes its current Information State (I). Based on the new knowledge, it adjusts its trajectory to coordinate (X2, Y2). The same approach is used to get to the future coordinates. The first step in carrying it out would be to model the information state. Every coordinate in the field is associated with one another since there are maxima and minima in the spatial field. This implies the existence of a normal distribution as well. Thus, as observed by Banerjee et al. [17], our perception of the world or our information state could be modelled under a Gaussian process. The graph below illustrates how variance causes some points to have extremely significant uncertainty and other cases to have very little uncertainty. The process's randomness will simulate the actual state in the world.

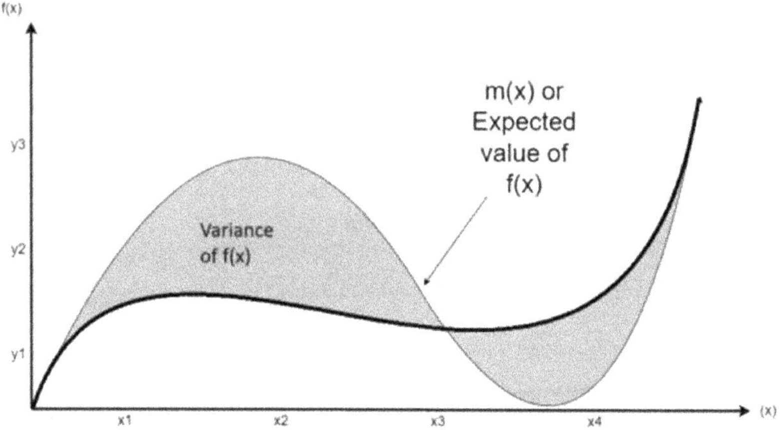

Figure 9. Initial Gaussian parameters.

The random variable $f(x)$ identifies each point x in the spatial field. For an ensemble of random variables in a Gaussian space, the mean and covariance function are given by,

$$\text{Meanorm}(x) = E[f(x)], \text{ where } E \text{ is the expected value of } f(x) \tag{3}$$

$$\text{Covariance or } k(x.x') = E[f(x) - m(x)\,(f(x') - m(x')] \tag{4}$$

Once a sensor retrieves new information at a specific coordinate, the information state (I) or Gaussian process is updated as follow:

$$f_{NEW}|X_{NEW}.X_{CURRENT}.f_{CURRENT} = \text{N (UpdatedMean.Updated Covariance)} \tag{5}$$

where f = Sample value and X = Sample location.

The updated mean is given by:

$$K(X_{NEW}.X_{CURRENT}).K(X_{CURRENT}.X_{CURRENT})^{-1}.f \tag{6}$$

The updated covariance is given by:

$$K(X_{NEW}.X_{NEW}) - K(X_{NEW}.X_{CURRENT}).K(X_{CURRENT}.X_{CURRENT})^{-1} \\ K(X_{CURRENT}.X_{NEW}) \tag{7}$$

Visually, the variance is shown to decrease while the mean is moved on the graph. This is how the sensor-gathered new data from the outside environment used it to update the information state. Additionally, it should be highlighted that the new information state only depends on the sample location and is mutually exclusive with the sample value.

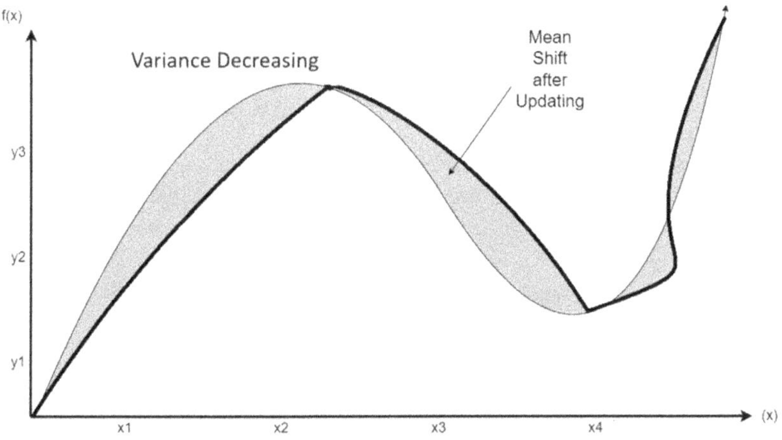

Figure 10. Updated Gaussian parameters

The mean and covariance functions are sufficient to define a Gaussian process. But would it be enough to define the information state? Sometimes we may not know the depth profile or whether the concentration levels at two different points are correlated or not. This will create a hurdle in defining the mean and covariance functions to be chosen.

Hence, in order to counter this, an appropriate strategy would be to create a model of the covariance itself. According to Murray et al. [18], selecting proper hyper parameters may allow us to do so. Examples of such hyper parameters are the Covariate Matrix $\{M\}$, $\sigma^2{}_{f,}\sigma^2{}_n$ or θ. The parameterised covariance function would look like,

$$k(x_A, x_B) = \sigma_f^2 \exp\left(-\frac{1}{2}(x_A - x_B)^T M(x_A - x_B)\right) + \sigma_n^2 \delta_{AB} \tag{8}$$

Now that we've created a strategy for updating the information state, we need to recognise an acquisition function that determines the location for the next sampling. This function would be defined over the interest space and would assess how well that place would be suited for sampling. This allows us to set a threshold and sample at a position where the function is maximised.

Depending on the conditions, different kinds of acquisition functions can be applied. We may only need to lessen the uncertainty in our information state in some circumstances. The optimal function for this circumstance would be Entropy or Variance [19]. It is given by.

$$h(x) = (k(x, x))^{1/2} \tag{9}$$

In other cases where finding the deepest point (or maxima/minima) is the priority, we could use a Mean and Variance acquisition function.

$$h(x) = m(x) + a(k(x, x))^{1/2} \tag{10}$$

The Mutual Information should be taken into consideration as another acquisition function. In this instance, we give more significance to the requirement that the sample location should not only be favourable overall but also best for retrieving information from adjacent locations.

The final stage of the algorithm must consider the termination criteria. Once we have reached a point of information saturation, it is possible to see that the hyperparameters responsible for defining the model's uncertainty have peaked and the algorithm has terminated. Sample exhaustion is a further criterion that can be identified by the development of relatively few new samples in the following cycles. Finally, if the variance is inside a "tolerance bound" where its error is at a minimum, the requirement might be satisfied.

2.3.2 Parallel Computing for Efficient Data Transformation

We now examine methods for reducing the amount of time and processing power needed for the data transformation and extraction stage. The obtained data is heterogeneous in nature and hence has to be transformed and put on a data warehouse for supervised learning. Parallel processing using the Map Reduce approach is suggested by Stonebraker et al. [20] for such scenarios. The vast amount of data is initially split into several sub processes of manageable volume. The "Map" step is responsible for data normalization while the "Reduce" step is used for aggregation.

When allocating a set of equally split tuples (T_n) into S segments, each tuple in the data is assigned the (N mod S) condition. So, if there are three segments, the first, fourth, and seventh tuples are in the first collection, while the second, fifth, and eighth tuples are in the next collection, and so on. This is labelled as the Round Robin approach.

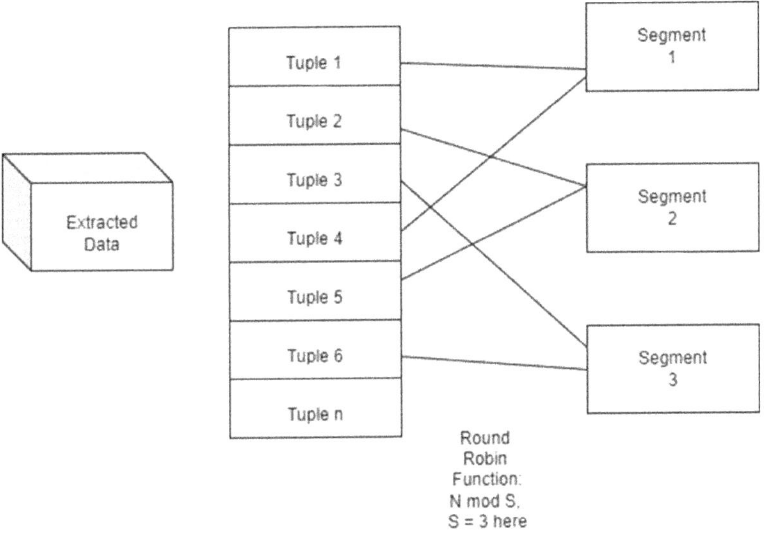

Figure 11. Round Robin segmentation

The segments in this example are workstations with capable processors, each of which serves as a file system. Each of these file systems is linked to the others. This defines a distributed file system, also known as DFS. Once the data is segmented, there is no further data movement and the mapping function is supplied to each of these workstations. This is for the purpose of reduced server latency [21]. The distributed system is under the supervision of a central controller.

There is potential for a network partition when generating the key-value pair, in which case the link between the systems is lost. In that case, it is up to the central controller to restart the process. For this to work, both the map and reduce functions must be idempotent, which means that their output must be consistent regardless of how many times they are invoked.

In the following example, there are two sections with input files containing health-related measurements. The mapping function's objective is to assign key-value pairs to multiple equally large data chunks. It looks for each of these metrics in a file and calculates the frequency of occurrence for each word. The frequency is designated as the value, whereas the key is designated as the word. The key-value pair is then shuffled by accumulating the sets of all the key value pairs from various input files. This facilitates the process of classifying them according to reduction. In the reduction stage, we group some of these data pieces into a single category if they share a similar key.

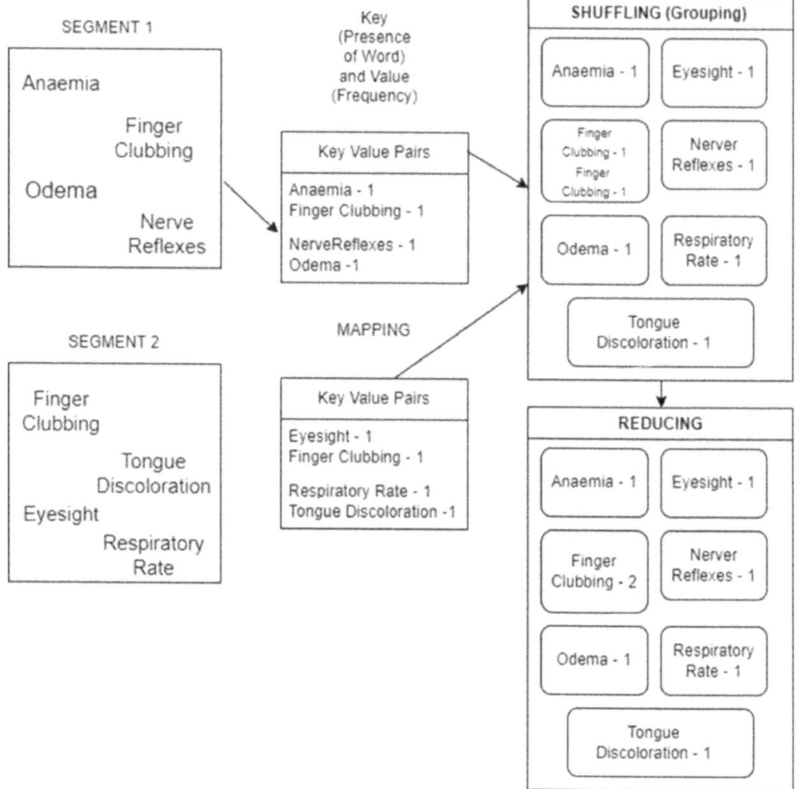

Figure 12. Mapping and reducing workflow

To quantify the improvement, we examine the parallel efficiency of Map-Reduce. Let $\sigma D_{ORIGINAL}$ be the data collected after the mapping phase and W. $D_{ORIGINAL}$ be the net amount of actual work to be done, where W can be any parametric number and does not have to be a constant. The overhead is now calculated as $\frac{\sigma D_{ORIGINAL}}{P}$ where P is the number of processors in use. This is the data that each mapper writes for an input file.

Each reducer must read this data before beginning the reduce procedure. So it must read $(1/P)^{th}$ of the data from each mapper and from P separate mappers.

Hence, Communication Time required by

$$\text{Reducer} = \frac{1}{P}.P.\left(\frac{\sigma D_{ORIGINAL}}{P}\right) \text{ or } \frac{\sigma D_{ORIGINAL}}{P} \tag{11}$$

The total overhead is the sum of the above values. The parallel efficiency is thus given by [24].

$$E = \left(\frac{\text{Expected Work Done}}{\text{No. of Processors ((Work Done per processor)} + 2C * \text{Total Overhead)}} \right)$$

Or $$E = \left(\frac{wD}{p\left(\left(\frac{wD}{P}\right) + 2C\,\frac{\sigma D_{ORIGINAL}}{P}\right)} \right) = \frac{1}{1 + \left(\frac{2C}{w}\right)\sigma} \tag{12}$$

As a result, because the value is independent of P, it demonstrates that the map reduction process is scalable and that huge efficiency can be attained without the need for high-performance processors.

It is, however, reliant on W. As the useful work per processor grows, the efficiency approaches one.

For enhanced efficiency, the additional data produced following the map step (σ) must also be reduced. Combiners can be employed to prevent data from being blown up after the map phase. To confirm the preceding statement, Kavitha et al. [22] demonstrate the same in a practical environment.

Thus, it can be said that the ETL paradigm is optimized greatly through parallel computing. Following the Data Transformation phase, we move on to discuss the use of deep learning for predictive disease diagnosis on the data.

3. Case Studies of Deep Learning for Disease Diagnosis

The final step in predictive disease diagnosis is the use of deep learning (DL) algorithms. They are different from conventional machine learning algorithms since their extracted data can take several forms, including metric measurements, written prescriptions, and image scans. Valentina Emilia Balas et al. [25] emphasize the importance of obtaining appropriate knowledge on the prerequisites for diagnosing a certain condition in order to comprehend its application.

In order to understand how this works, let's have a look at how a straightforward metric measurement such as the heart response rate can be utilised to detect hypopnoea or apnoea occurrences in patients with underlying Parkinson's disease [26]. Motor symptoms are those that have an impact on balance, flexibility, and movement. Deterioration of posture and reactive responses, tight muscles due to delayed nerve signals, increasing freezing, and gait arrest are all indications of this illness.

In terms of the ease of the data obtained, detecting these symptoms is highly challenging. According to Braak's theory [27], it is simpler to diagnose the non-motor symptoms that come before these motor symptoms. These include monitoring sleep disruptions or keeping track of nervous system disorders through

IoT devices. Other major health risks, including COVID19, are also characterised by non-motor symptoms as loss of smell, headaches, and muscular and head pain. Let's now demonstrate how a prediction system can be created by training a model with these symptoms with help of several case studies.

Rui Zhao et al. [28] propose a method of retrieving hierarchical information through deep learning. This is significant since it would allow us to extrapolate many symptoms by putting them through neural networks with nonlinear layers. Linear neural networks behave similarly to linear functions of the form y = mx + c, with y is increasing at a constant "rate" with respect to x. Non-linear neural networks operate on the same idea as non-linear functions with a variable rate of change and are capable of handling diverse data. Henry Friday et al. [30] developed a generative model used on data gathered by wearable devices responsible for automatically capturing data. It implemented use of auto encoder and Restricted Boltzmann Machine in order to generate predictions.

Nonlinear neural networks rely on activation functions, layer convolution, or pooling. In the case of a certain scenario, the appropriate action can be taken. If many physiological parameters contribute to a single output, a pooling layer could be used to summarise the data using max/min or average functions. Convolution layers can be applied to a localized portion of a medical image to identify a local spot, such as lesion identification for early breast cancer. Finally, activation functions work with sigmoid or relu functions to improve model training and introduce nonlinearity.

The Boltzmann Machine Technique is applied across both case studies, which is commonly used to describe binary data [29]. It works by assigning a probability to each potential binary vector in order to calculate the likelihood of other vectors belonging to the same distribution. It is especially useful for binary data, where a specific set of values denotes the presence of a feature, and for monitoring odd behaviours. For models with several distributions, the posterior probability of a specific distribution yielding the desired results is given by.

$$P(\text{Model } i|\text{data}) = \frac{p(\text{data}|\text{Model } i)}{\Sigma_n p(\text{data}|\text{Model } j)} \tag{13}$$

Data for any model is created in two processes, one after the other. We begin by identifying the hidden states in the prior distribution. The visible states emerge conditionally from these hidden states. As a result, the likelihood of a visible vector is calculated by adding all recognised hidden states.

$$\text{P}(v) = \sum_h p(h)p(v \mid h) \tag{14}$$

However, a new measurement is factored in a Boltzmann Machine, which is the energy between the configuration between the hidden and visible states, which is reliant on the probability in two ways. This is beneficial when the weights in a given distribution are varied. Let us take the following scenario for example:

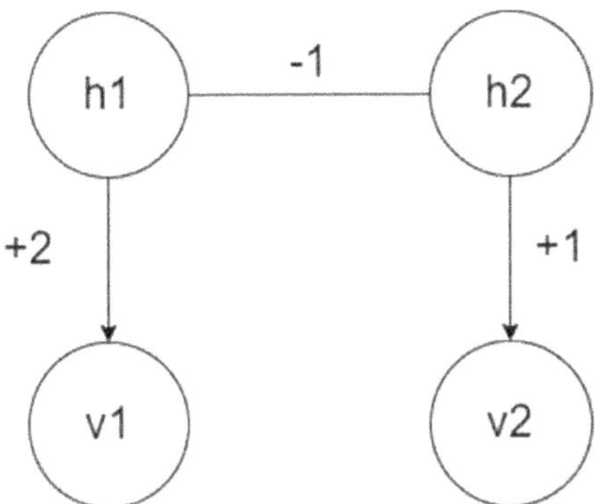

Figure 13. Illustration of weights in a distribution

Let the weight between hidden states (h1) and h2 be –1, the weight between h1 and v1 be +2, and the weight between h2 and v2 be +1. For the weight to be considered, both endpoints of a link must be binary values of 1.

e^{-E} provides the energy of a combined contribution. The likelihood or probability is calculated by dividing the energy of that configuration by the sum of all conceivable combinations. It is given by

$$P = e^{-E} \Big/ \sum e^{-E} \tag{15}$$

To understand this better, see Table 1.

However, because the number of hidden states is exponential, there is a rise in processing time and observed over-fitting, as Huang et al. [31] indicate. As a result, the Markov Chain Monte Carlo is particularly beneficial for reducing both over-fitting and uncertainty of sampling. Through this method, we are trying to obtain a finite set of samples, whose function is to analyze the range of possible outcomes and spent equivalent time in each interval, proportional to the distribution's density. Let's look at a straightforward MRI where we need to calculate the tumour's ratio to a certain region of the brain in order to better grasp the Markov Chain Monte Carlo method.

Here, random locations in space have been selected where X ~ U [Xmin, Xmax] whereas Y ~ U [Ymin, Ymax]. The points inside the tumour region are then classified as N_{INSIDE}, and the points outside the region as $N_{OUTSIDE}$. This process is repeated iteratively until $N_{INSIDE}/(N_{INSIDE} + N_{OUTSIDE})$ is precise and doesn't change much across future iterations.

The future state of a Markov Chain should be reliant on the current state. As a result, the probability of the next point in the region is provided by

$$P(p_{next} \in \text{Tumour} \mid p_{current} \in \text{Tumour}) = (N_{INSIDE} - 1)/(N_{INSIDE} + N_{OUTSIDE} - 1) \tag{16}$$

Additionally, the probability of the next point not lying in region is given by

$$P(p_{next} \in \text{Tumour} \mid p_{current} \notin \text{Tumour}) = (N_{INSIDE})/(N_{INSIDE} + N_{OUTSIDE} - 1) \tag{17}$$

Table 1. Possible scenarios of Energy allocation among hidden and visible states.

Visible State (v1)	Visible State (v2)	Hidden State (h1)	Hidden State (h2)	–E	e^{-E}
1	1	1	1	–1 (Between Hidden States h1 and h2) +2 (Between Hidden State h1 and Visible State v1) +1 (Between Hidden State h2 and Visible State v2) = +2	7.39
1	1	1	0	+2 (Between Hidden State h1 and Visible State v1) The hidden state h2 doesn't exist and so doesn't v2.	7.39
1	1	0	1	+1 (Between Hidden State h2 and Visible State v2) The hidden state h1 doesn't exist and so doesn't v1.	2.72
1	1	0	0	0	1
1	0	1	1	–1 (Between Hidden States h1 and h2) +2 (Between Hidden State h1 and Visible State v1) = +1	2.72
1	0	1	0	+2 (Between Hidden State h1 and Visible State v1)	7.39
1	0	0	1	0	1
1	0	0	0	0	1
0	1	1	1	0	1
0	1	1	0	0	1
0	1	0	1	+1 (Between Hidden State h2 and Visible State v2)	2.72
0	1	0	0	0	1
0	0	1	1	–1 (Between Hidden States h1 and h2)	0.37
0	0	1	0	0	1
0	0	0	1	0	1
0	0	0	0	0	1
Summation of $e^{-E} = 39.70$					

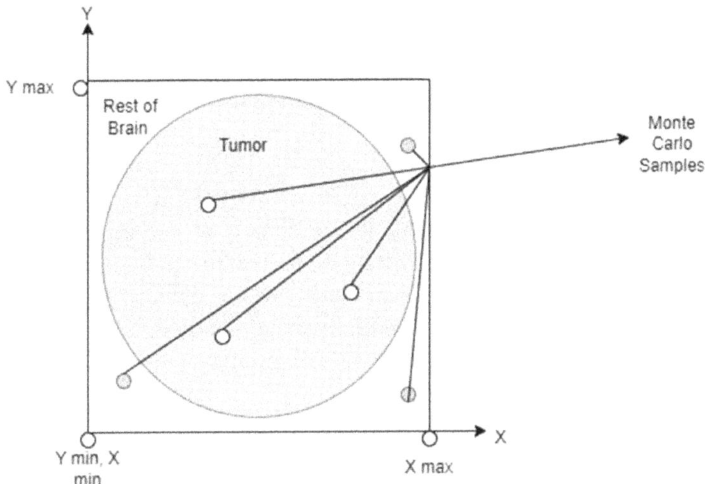

Figure 14. Monte Carlo space selection

It is feasible to generate Markov Chains using these two probabilities, starting with a random initial point that can be either inside (p_{INSIDE}) or outside ($p_{OUTSIDE}$). The probabilities given above are used to generate the following state. This is repeated until we have an entire chain of states. It can be observed that regardless of the random start, all chains eventually converge to be identical. According to Brockwell et al. [33], these chains can be successfully executed in parallel to save processing time. As a result, the techniques described above can be used to detect anomalies in metric measurements while interpreting them as binary vectors or in medical imaging.

Let's examine a few more medical issues where deep learning algorithms have been used for diagnosis . A contemporary method for studying hormonal instability through the assessment of endocrine glands and growing-age developmental difficulties due to hereditary reasons is bone density examination [34].

With the use of a CT scan, the patient's left ventricle is radiologically assessed using the Tanmer-Whitehouse (TW) method. Reconstructing the image is one of the crucial processes, and the CNN architecture's de-noising capacity is essentially required. In nature, noise is a random inaccuracy that may be seen in the RGB values of individual pixels in an image. Traditional algorithms sometimes assume that an image's "noise" is a homogeneous Gaussian distribution whereas in fact "Blind/Real" noise is more complex. To combat it, Zhao et al. [35] suggest a pyramidal step-by-step architecture. This consists of several modules.

The first module is necessary to add weights for better representation. The input (I) has been divided into a number of channels. Each channel has a weight assigned to it. The attention or "weights" are managed by the first module. The entire number of channels, N, makes up the size of the vector in which the set of weights is kept. The input is sent through this vector. The machine learning algorithm needs to be trained in order to learn the weight distribution. This is accomplished by first implementing a Global Average Pooling layer, then implementing the ReLu and Sigmoid activation functions, respectively.

4. Conclusion

The output is then sent through numerous kernels of varying sizes for down sampling. This is notably effective for accumulating enough information to perform recognition efficiently in even low-resolution photos [36]. Each of these kernels modified variants is subjected to average pooling. Finally, the image is reconstructed to the same size by up sampling after being done several times with different kernel sizes.

According to Li et al. [37], the receptive space for artificial neurons in a neural network is often configured to share a constant size. Because there are various kernel size versions in the proposed unit for selected kernels, a softmax activation function is supplied to concatenate them all in our module with the help of the present attention or information. When it comes to intricate denoising, this strategy has been proven to offer optimal solutions.

Hence, it can be concluded that the traditional methods of feature prediction and image analysis observed in healthcare have had a few efficient innovative methods in recent years, which can look to build a foundation for further improvement.

References

[1] Gehlot, A. and Misra, N. An IoT based smart healthcare medical system using deep learning algorithm. 2022 IEEE 2nd Mysore Sub Section International Conference (MysuruCon), Mysuru, India, pp. 1-6, 2022, doi: 10.1109/MysuruCon55714.2022.9972370.

[2] Engel, V.J.L. and Supangkat, S.H. Context-aware inference model for cold-chain logistics monitoring. 2014 International Conference on ICT For Smart Society (ICISS), Bandung, Indonesia, pp. 192-196, 2014, doi: 10.1109/ICTSS.2014.7013172.

[3] Kang, J.J., Dibaei, M., Luo, G., Yang, W., Haskell-Dowland, P. et al. An energy-efficient and secure data inference framework for internet of health things: A pilot study. Sensors, 21(1):312, 2021, https://doi.org/10.3390/s21010312.

[4] Elshrkawey, M., Elsherif, S.M. and Elsayed Wahed, M. An enhancement approach for reducing the energy consumption in wireless sensor networks. Journal of King Saud University - Computer and Information Sciences [online] 30(2): 259–267, 2018, doi:https://doi.org/10.1016/j.jksuci.2017.04.002.

[5] Hämäläinen, J., Jauhiainen, S. and Kärkkäinen, T. Comparison of internal clustering validation indices for prototype-based clustering. Algorithms, 10(3): 105. 2017), doi:https://doi.org/10.3390/a10030105.

[6] Tiwari, T. and Nihar Ranjan Roy. Heirarchical Clustering in Heterogeneous Wireless Sensor Networks: A Survey. 2015. doi:https://doi.org/10.1109/ccaa.2015.7148596.

[7] Kim, J.-M., Park, S.-H., Han, Y.-J. and Chung, T.-M. CHEF: Cluster head election mechanism using fuzzy logic in wireless sensor networks. 10th International Conference on Advanced Communication Technology, Feb. 2008, https://doi.org/10.1109/icact.2008.4493846.

[8] Diamant, Roee, and Lutz Lampe. Spatial Reuse Time-Division Multiple Access for Broadcast Ad Hoc Underwater Acoustic Communication Networks. 36(2): 172–185, 12 May 2011, https://doi.org/10.1109/joe.2011.2107950.

[9] Hadded, Mohamed, Paul Mühlethaler, Anis Laouiti, Rachid Zagrouba and Leila Azouz Saidane. TDMA-based MAC protocols for vehicular ad hoc networks: a survey, qualitative analysis, and open research issues. IEEE Communications Surveys & Tutorials, 17(4): 2461-2492, 2015, hal.science/hal-01211437v1/document, https://doi.org/10.1109/comst.2015.2440374.

[10] Nagpurkar, A.W. and Jaiswal, S.K. An overview of WSN and RFID network integration. 2015 2nd International Conference on Electronics and Communication Systems (ICECS), Coimbatore, India, pp. 497-502, 2015, doi: 10.1109/ECS.2015.7124956.

[11] Muhammad Sadiq, Nordiana Binti Ahmed and Ely Salvana. Design and testing of an epidermal RFID mechanism in a smart indoor human tracking system. IEEE Sensors Journal, 21(4): 5476–5486, 15 Feb. 2021, https://doi.org/10.1109/jsen.2020.3036233.

[12] Yang, Yahui, Wu, Yujie, Xia, Min, Qin, Zhijing et al. (2009). A RFID Network Planning Method Based on Genetic Algorithm. Networks Security, Wireless Communications and Trusted Computing, International Conference. 534-537. 10.1109/NSWCTC.2009.238.

[13] Haupt, R.L. Optimum population size and mutation rate for a simple real genetic algorithm that optimizes array factors. IEEE Antennas and Propagation Society International Symposium. Transmitting Waves of Progress to the Next Millennium. 2000 Digest. Held in conjunction with: USNC/URSI National Radio Science Meeting. C, Salt Lake City, UT, USA, vol. 2, pp. 1034-1037, 2000, doi: 10.1109/APS.2000.875398.

[14] Hassanat, Ahmad, Khalid Almohammadi, Esra Alkafaween, Eman Abunavas, Awni Hammouri and Suryaprakash, V.B. Choosing mutation and crossover ratios for genetic algorithms—A review with a new dynamic approach. *Information*, 10(12): 390, 10 Dec. 2019, https://doi.org/10.3390/info10120390.

[15] Gong, Yue-Jiao, Shen, Meie, Zhang, Jun, Kaynak, Okyay, Chen, Wei-neng and Zhan, Zhi-Hui. Optimizing RFID network planning by using a particle swarm optimization algorithm with redundant reader elimination. IEEE Transactions on Industrial Informatics, 8(4): 900–912, Nov. 2012, https://doi.org/10.1109/tii.2012.2205390. Accessed 16 Mar. 2022.

[16] Gedik, B., Ling, L. and Philip, S.L. ASAP: An adaptive sampling approach to data collection in sensor networks. IEEE Transactions on Parallel and Distributed Systems, 18(12): 1766-1783, Dec. 2007, https://doi.org/10.1109/tpds.2007.1110.

[17] Banerjee, Onureena, Laurent El Ghaoui, and Alexandre D'Aspremont. Model Selection through Sparse Maximum Likelihood Estimation for Multivariate Gaussian or Binary Data. 9(15): 485-516, 1 June 2008, https://doi.org/10.1145/1390681.1390696.

[18] Murray, Iain, and Ryan P. Adams. Slice sampling covariance hyperparameters of latent gaussian models. ArXiv (Cornell University), 4 June 2010.
[19] José Miguel Hernández-Lobato, Michael A. Gelbart, Matthew W. Hoffman, Ryan P. Adams and Zoubin Ghahramani. Predictive entropy search for bayesian optimization with unknown constraints. International Conference on Machine Learning, 1699-1707, 6 July 2015.
[20] Stonebraker, Michael, Daniel Abadi, David J. DeWitt, Sam Madden, Erik Paulson, Andrew Pavlo et al. Map reduce and parallel DBMSs. Communications of the ACM, 53(1): 64-71, Jan. 2010, https://doi.org/10.1145/1629175.1629197. Accessed 4 June 2020.
[21] Jadhav, Prof. Ashvini. Fast file downloading using network coding in distributed system. International Journal of Engineering and Computer Science, 20 Aug. 2016, https://doi.org/10.18535/ijecs/v4i11.07.
[22] C. Kavitha, S.R. Srividhya, Wen Cheng Lai and Vinodhini Mani. IMapC: Inner MAPping combiner to enhance the performance of MapReduce in Hadoop. Electronics, 11(10): 1599-1599, 17 May 2022, https://doi.org/10.3390/electronics11101599.
[23] Shifeng Fang, Li Da Xu, Yunqiang Zhu, Jiaerheng Ahati, Huan Pei and Jianwu Yan. An integrated system for regional environmental monitoring and management based on Internet of Things. IEEE Transactions on Industrial Informatics, 10(2): 1596-1605, May 2014, https://doi.org/10.1109/tii.2014.2302638.
[24] Kao, Chiang. Efficiency measurement for parallel production systems. European Journal of Operational Research, 196(3): 1107-1112, Aug. 2009, https://doi.org/10.1016/j.ejor.2008.04.020.
[25] Valentina Emilia Balas, Sanjiban Sekhar Roy, Pijush Samui and Sharma, D. Handbook of Deep Learning Applications. Cham, Springer International Publishing, 2019.
[26] Yoshino, K., Kawaguchi, A., Yata, S., Iyama, A. and Sakoda, S. Analysis of heart rate response to obstructive Apnea/Hypopnea events in patients with parkinson's disease with relatively severe sleep Apnea Syndrome. Informatics in Medicine Unlocked, 23: 100554, 2021, https://doi.org/10.1016/j.imu.2021.100554.
[27] Konings, B., Villatoro, L., Van den Eynde, J., Barhona, G., Burns, R. and McKnight, M. Gastrointestinal syndromes preceding a diagnosis of Parkinson's disease: Testing Braak's hypothesis using a nationwide database for comparison with Alzheimer's disease and cerebrovascular diseases. doi: 10.1136/gutjnl-2023-329685.
[28] Rui Zhao, Ruqaing Yan, Zhenghua Chen, Kezhi Mao, Peng Wang and Robert Gao. Deep learning and its applications to machine health monitoring: A survey. Mechanical Systems and Signal Processing, 14(8), Aug. 2015.
[29] Salakhutdinov, Ruslan and Geoffrey Hinton. An efficient learning procedure for deep boltzmann machines. Neural Computation, 24(8): 1967-2006, Aug. 2012, https://doi.org/10.1162/neco_a_00311.
[30] Nweke, Henry Friday. Deep learning algorithms for human activity recognition using mobile and wearable sensor networks: State of the art and research challenges. Expert Systems with Applications, 105: 233-261, Sept. 2018, www.sciencedirect.com/science/article/pii/S0957417418302136, https://doi.org/10.1016/j.eswa.2018.03.056.

[31] Huang, Gao, Zhuang Liu, Laurens van der Maaten and Kilian Q. Weinberger. Densely Connected Convolutional Networks. 2017 IEEE Conference on Computer Vision and Pattern Recognition (CVPR), pp. 2261-2269, July 2017, https://doi.org/10.1109/cvpr.2017.243.

[32] Williamson, S., Dubey, A. and Xing, E. Parallel Markov Chain Monte Carlo for nonparametric mixture models. International Conference on Machine Learning, 28(1): 98-106, 16 June 2013.

[33] Brockwell, Anthony. Parallel Markov Chain Monte Carlo simulation by pre-fetching. Journal of Computational and Graphical Statistics, 15(1): 246-261, 1 Mar. 2006, https://doi.org/10.1198/106186006x100579.

[34] Bellot, P., de Los Campos, G. and Pérez-Enciso, M. Can deep learning improve genomic prediction of complex human traits? Genetics, 210(3): 809-819, 31 Aug. 2018, https://doi.org/10.1534/genetics.118.301298.

[35] Zhao, Yiyun, Zhuqing Jiang, Aidong Men and Guodong Ju. Pyramid real image denoising network. 2019 IEEE Visual Communications and Image Processing (VCIP), Dec. 2019, https://doi.org/10.1109/vcip47243.2019.8965754.

[36] Xu, Yong and Zhong Jin. Down-Sampling Face Images and Low-Resolution Face Recognition. 1 Jan. 2008, https://doi.org/10.1109/icicic.2008.234.

[37] Xiang Li, Wenhai Wang, Xiaolin Hu and Jian Yang. Selective Kernel Networks. Computer Vision Foundation, Jan. 2019.

CHAPTER

5

Transforming Healthcare through Machine Learning and the Internet of Things

Faridoddin Shariaty*

Institute of Electronics and Telecommunications, Peter the Great St. Petersburg Polytechnic University, Saint-Petersburg, Russia

Machine learning (ML) and the Internet of Things (IoT) are two of the most influential and disruptive technologies in the modern world. They have the potential to transform healthcare by providing innovative solutions that can improve the quality, efficiency, accessibility, affordability, and safety of healthcare services. In this chapter, we explore the current and future applications of ML and IoT in healthcare. Additionally, the challenges and considerations that need to be addressed to ensure their ethical, legal, and social implications are handled appropriately. We review some of the most important applications of ML in healthcare, such as disease diagnosis and predictive analytics, personalized treatment plans, image analysis and radiology, and drug discovery. We also review some of the most promising applications of IoT in healthcare, such as remote patient monitoring, smart healthcare facilities, and medication management. Furthermore, we review some of the most exciting applications of ML and IoT in healthcare that leverage their combined capabilities, such as early warning systems, predictive maintenance, and patient-centred care. Additionally, we review some of the most critical challenges and considerations for ML and IoT in healthcare that involve addressing their data privacy and security, data quality and standardization, integration and interoperability, and ethical and regulatory issues. Finally, we review some of the most potential future directions for ML and IoT in healthcare that involve developing AI-powered virtual health assistants, population health management systems, and

*Corresponding author: shariaty3@gmail.com

drug personalization methods. We hope that this chapter will provide you with a comprehensive overview of the current state-of-the-art and future trends of ML and IoT in healthcare, as well as inspire you to explore further research opportunities and practical applications in this domain.

1. Introduction

Machine learning (ML) and the Internet of Things (IoT) are two of the most influential and disruptive technologies in the modern world. ML is a field of artificial intelligence that involves the design of algorithms that enable computer systems to learn and make predictions or decisions based on data. IoT is a network of interconnected devices and sensors that collect, communicate, and share data over the internet. Together, ML and IoT can create powerful applications that can transform various domains and industries, such as healthcare. Healthcare is a domain that faces many challenges and opportunities in the 21st century, such as increasing demand, rising costs, aging populations, chronic diseases, pandemics, and health disparities. Healthcare also generates and consumes vast amounts of data from various sources, such as electronic health records, medical images, laboratory tests, wearable devices, and online platforms. ML and IoT can help address these challenges and opportunities by providing innovative solutions that can improve the quality, efficiency, accessibility, affordability, and safety of healthcare services [1-3].

We will discuss the following topics in this chapter (Figure 1):

1. Machine Learning in Healthcare: We will review some of the most important applications of ML in healthcare, such as disease diagnosis and predictive analytics, personalized treatment plans, image analysis and radiology, and drug discovery [4].
2. The Internet of Things in Healthcare: Some of the most promising applications of IoT in healthcare have been reviewed, such as remote patient monitoring, smart healthcare facilities, and medication management.
3. Synergies between Machine Learning and IoT in Healthcare: some of the most exciting applications of ML and IoT in healthcare have been reviewed that leverage their combined capabilities, such as early warning systems, predictive maintenance, and patient-centred care.
4. Challenges and Considerations: Some of the most critical challenges and considerations for ML and IoT in healthcare have been reviewed that involve addressing data privacy and security, data quality and standardization, integration and interoperability, ethical and regulatory issues.
5. Future Directions: Some of the most potential future directions for ML and IoT in healthcare that involve developing AI-powered virtual health assistants, population health management systems, and drug personalization methods have been reviewed.

We hope that this chapter will provide you with a comprehensive overview of the current state-of-the-art and future trends of ML and IoT in healthcare and inspire you to explore further research opportunities and practical applications in this domain.

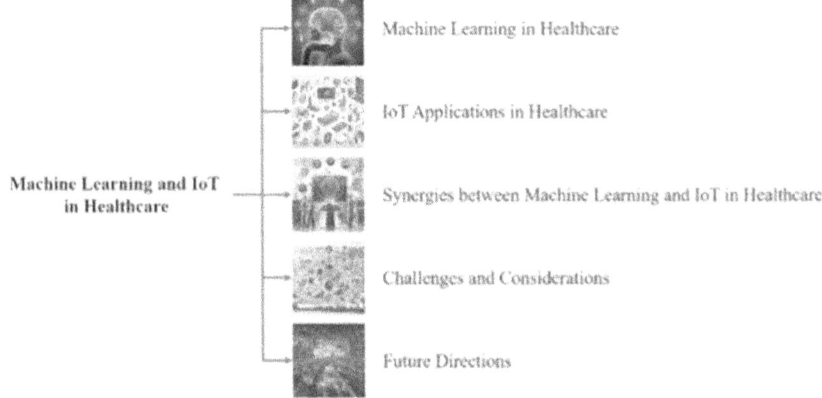

Figure 1. The overall theme of ML and IoT powered healthcare system

2. Machine Learning in Healthcare

As a branch of artificial intelligence, machine learning refers to the creation of algorithms that let computer systems learn and make predictions or decisions based on data. In healthcare, ML has emerged as a powerful tool for extracting valuable insights from vast and complex datasets. Machine learning has many applications in healthcare, such as diagnosis, prognosis, treatment, prevention, monitoring, and management of diseases and health conditions [5].

2.1 Disease Diagnosis and Predictive Analytics

Predictive analytics and illness diagnosis are two of the most significant uses of machine learning in healthcare. Machine learning can help diagnose various diseases and health conditions based on the symptoms, signs, tests, and images of the patients. Machine learning can also help predict the risk, progression, and outcome of diseases and associated health conditions based on the historical and current data of the patients. Some examples of disease diagnosis and predictive analytics using machine learning are:

2.1.1 Diabetes

Machine learning can help diagnose diabetes and prediabetes based on the blood glucose levels, blood pressure, body mass index, age, gender, and family history of the patients [6]. The process involves utilizing models like

Artificial Neural Networks (ANN) or Deep Neural Networks (DNN) that can learn and recognize complex patterns within patient data. For instance, an ANN could analyse extensive datasets of patient information, searching for intricate relationships between various factors and diabetes diagnosis. The model fine-tunes its parameters through a learning process to make accurate predictions. The predictive aspect involves leveraging mathematical equations and statistical methods to estimate the risk of complications and mortality in diabetes patients. These predictions often incorporate multiple variables, such as glycated haemoglobin levels, kidney function, cardiovascular status, and other critical factors [7, 8].

Figure 2 Illustrates a neural network model designed for diabetes diagnosis, which predicts whether an individual is healthy (labeled as "1," indicating the absence of diabetes) or sick (labeled as "0," signifying the presence of diabetes). The network consists of three hidden layers, which play a crucial role in extracting and learning intricate patterns and relationships within the input data to make accurate predictions [9].

Input Layer: The input layer serves as the initial point of the neural network, representing the features or variables used for diabetes diagnosis. The input layer is responsible for receiving and passing the input features (X) to the first hidden layer of the neural network. Each feature is denoted as X_i, where i represents the specific feature. For example, the input for "Pregnancies" (X_1) would be the number of pregnancies. These features include the following [10]:

- **Pregnancies:** The number of pregnancies.
- **PG Concentration:** Plasma glucose concentration measured after 2 hours during an oral glucose tolerance test.
- **Diastolic BP:** Diastolic Blood Pressure in millimeters of mercury (mm Hg).
- **Tri Fold Thick:** Triceps Skin Fold Thickness in millimeters (mm).
- **Serum Ins:** 2-Hour Serum Insulin measured in micro international units per milliliter (mu U/ml).
- **BMI:** Body Mass Index, calculated as weight in kilograms divided by the square of height in meters.
- **DP Function:** The Diabetes Pedigree Function, a genetic measure of diabetes.
- **Age:** The age of the individual in years.

Hidden Layers (3 layers): The three hidden layers are the core of the neural network, responsible for processing the input data and learning complex relationships among the variables. These layers consist of nodes (neurons) that perform mathematical computations on the input data, transforming it into a format that is suitable for the final prediction. In the hidden layers, the neural network performs several essential mathematical operations:

1. **Linear Combination:** Each neuron (node) in the hidden layer calculates a weighted sum of the inputs from the previous layer, applies an activation

function, and passes the result to the next layer. The weighted sum (Z) for a neuron is calculated as follows:

$$Z_\mathrm{i} = \sum_{j=1}^{n} (W_{(ij)}.X_j) + b_{(i)} \tag{1}$$

Z_i: Weighted sum for neuron i.
W_{ij}: Weight connecting neuron i to input feature j.
X_j: Value of input feature j.
b_i: Bias term for neuron i.

2. **Activation Function:** To add non-linearity to the network, the weighted sum (Z_i) is then passed via an activation function (F). The hyperbolic tangent function, rectified linear unit (ReLU), and sigmoid function are examples of common activation functions. One way to depict the activation function is as follows:

$$A_i = F(Z_i) \tag{2}$$

A_i: Activation of neuron i.

3. **Output of Hidden Layer:** The output of each neuron in the hidden layer becomes the input for neurons in the subsequent hidden layer or the output layer. The output of a hidden layer neuron can be represented as:

$$X^{(l)} = A \tag{3}$$

$X^{(l)}$: Output of the l-th layer.
A: Activation values from all neurons in the current layer.

Output Layer: In the output layer, the neural network processes the data to provide the final prediction. For binary classification tasks like disease diagnosis, the output layer typically employs the sigmoid function as the activation function. The sigmoid function maps values to the range [0, 1] and is often used to estimate the probability of belonging to one of the classes.

$$\hat{y} = \sigma(Z^{(\mathrm{out})}) \tag{4}$$

$\hat{y}$: Predicted output.
σ: Sigmoid activation function.
$Z^{(\mathrm{out})}$: Weighted sum of the final hidden layer.

The output of the sigmoid function, $\hat{y}$, represents the model's prediction regarding the individual's diabetic status. If $\hat{y}$ is close to 1, it indicates a prediction of being "Healthy," while if it is close to 0, it suggests a prediction of being "Sick."

The neural network processes the input data through its hidden layers, adjusting the internal weights and biases during training to optimize its predictive accuracy. As the data is propagated through the network, the model learns to recognize patterns and make predictions regarding the individual's diabetic status based on the input variables.

The model is trained by adjusting the weights (W_{ij}) and biases (b_i) through an iterative process called backpropagation to minimize the prediction error and enhance the model's accuracy. This training involves optimizing a loss function (typically cross-entropy for binary classification) using gradient descent. The three hidden layers are designed to capture and learn intricate patterns, allowing the neural network to provide accurate and reliable diabetes diagnosis results based on the features provided. Through an iterative training process, the network fine-tunes its internal parameters, ultimately enabling it to generalize from the training data and make predictions for new, unseen cases [11].

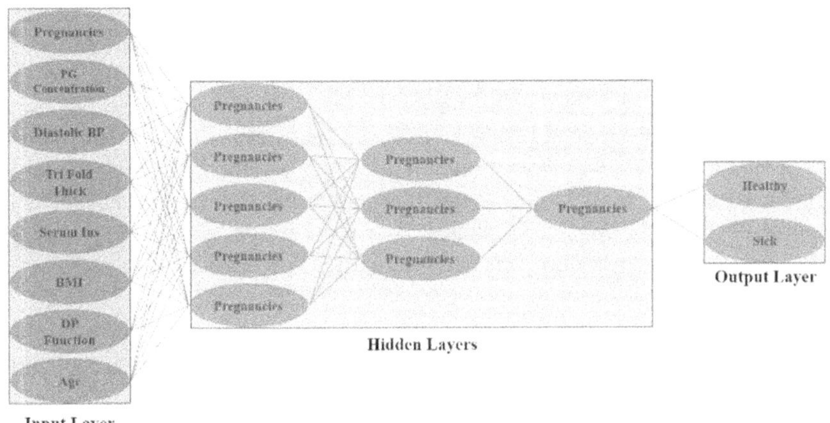

Figure 2. Simplified representation of an ANN for diabetes

2.1.2 Cancer

With the use of biopsy samples, gene expression profiles, imaging modalities, and clinical features, machine learning can assist in the diagnosis of a variety of cancers, including skin, brain, lung, and breast cancer. A common deep learning model for image analysis, including the interpretation of medical imaging like MRIs and X-rays, is called a convolutional neural network (CNN). CNNs employ a series of layers to automatically detect patterns and features in images, making them valuable for cancer diagnosis. Machine learning can also help predict the prognosis and survival of cancer patients based on the tumor stage, grade, size, location, molecular subtype, and treatment response of the patients. When predicting patient outcomes, survival analysis algorithms and equations play a significant role in estimating the likelihood of survival over a certain period [12-18].

Figure 3 illustrates a CNN architecture which serves as a powerful tool for the automated differentiation of COVID-19 symptoms from pulmonary edema in lung CT scans [19-21]. By leveraging deep learning techniques, it can extract and interpret intricate patterns and features within medical images, specifically CT scans of the lung. The key components of this CNN architecture include:

1. **Convolutional Layers:** The convolutional layers are responsible for scanning the input CT images with a set of learnable filters. These filters enable the network to detect various features and patterns, such as edges, textures, or specific shapes, within the images. This set works according to the following equation [22, 23]:

$$\text{Conv}(i,j) = \sum_{h=0}^{H-1}\sum_{w=0}^{W-1}\left[X(i+h,j+w)\cdot K(h,w)\right] \tag{5}$$

Conv(i, j): The output value at position (i, j) in the feature map.
$X(i + h, j + w)$: The input value at position $(i + h, j + w)$ in the input feature map.
$K(h, w)$: The weights of the convolutional filter at position (h, w).
H and W: The dimensions of the filter (height and width).

2. **ReLU Layer:** Rectified Linear Unit (ReLU) activation functions are applied after each convolution operation to introduce non-linearity into the model.
3. **Max Pooling:** Max pooling layers reduce the spatial dimensions of the data by selecting the maximum values from each region. This down sampling helps in retaining the most critical information while reducing computational complexity.
4. **Batch-Normalization Layers:** Batch normalization layers aim to stabilize and accelerate the training process by normalizing the inputs of the neural network:

$$\text{Batch\_Normalization }(x) = \gamma\cdot\left(\frac{x-\mu}{\sqrt{\sigma^2 \ +\varepsilon}}\right)+\beta \tag{6}$$

x: The input value to the batch normalization function.
γ: The scale parameter.
μ: The mean of the batch.
σ^2: The variance of the batch.
ε: A small constant to prevent division by zero.
β: The shift parameter.

5. **Fully Connected Layer:** The fully connected layer acts as a neural network classifier, making decisions based on the features extracted in the previous layers. It connects every neuron in the previous layer to every neuron in the current layer, allowing it to learn complex, non-local relationships between features.
6. **Dropout:** The dropout layer is used to prevent overfitting. During training, it randomly "drops out" (deactivates) a fraction of neurons, forcing the network to become more robust and generalize better.
7. **SoftMax Layer:** The SoftMax layer provides the final classification probabilities for the two conditions: COVID-19 symptoms and pulmonary edema. It ensures that the predicted probabilities sum up to one, making it clear which condition the model is leaning towards based on the input CT scan. SoftMax function for class i is calculated as below:

$$P(y = i|x) = \frac{e^{z_i}}{\sum_k e^{z_k}} \tag{7}$$

$P(y = i|x)$: The probability of class i given input x.
z_i: The weighted sum for class i.
e: The base of the natural logarithm.

The ultimate goal of this CNN architecture is to automatically classify lung CT scans into either COVID-19 symptoms or pulmonary edema. This enables healthcare professionals to make more informed and efficient decisions, particularly in critical situations, where rapid diagnosis is essential. The model's performance is achieved through a combination of image feature extraction, learned patterns, and neural network training, leading to accurate and timely differentiation between the two conditions.

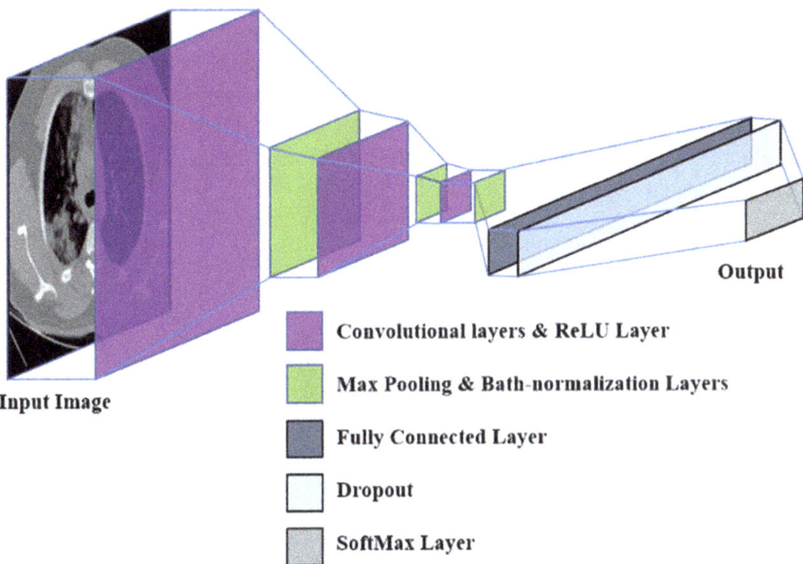

Figure 3. Convolutional Neural Network (CNN) for COVID-19 symptom differentiation

2.1.3 Cardiovascular Diseases

Using the patient's electrocardiogram (ECG), echocardiogram (ECHO), angiography, and other tests, machine learning can assist in the diagnosis of cardiovascular diseases such as coronary artery disease, heart failure, arrhythmia, and stroke. Various ML models, including decision trees and support vector machines, are utilized to analyse ECG data. These models consider various features extracted from ECG signals to identify irregularities associated with heart diseases. Moreover, predictive analytics for cardiovascular events, like myocardial infarction and cardiac arrest, involve statistical models and equations that factor in demographics, clinical data, genetics, and environmental variables. These equations often use survival analysis techniques to estimate the risk of adverse cardiovascular events over time.

Machine learning in disease diagnosis and predictive analytics has the potential to improve the accuracy, timeliness, and cost-effectiveness of healthcare services. However, there are many additional challenges and limitations that need to be addressed, such as data quality, privacy, security, ethics, regulation, interpretability, explainability, trustworthiness, and social impact. Therefore, it is important to develop machine learning methods that are robust, reliable, transparent, fair, accountable, and human-centred for disease diagnosis and predictive analytics applications.

2.2 Personalized Treatment Plans

Another important application of machine learning in healthcare is personalized treatment plans. Machine learning can help tailor medical interventions to the specific characteristics and preferences of each individual patient, such as their genetic makeup, lifestyle, environment, and medical history. Machine learning can also help optimize the dosage, timing, and combination of drugs and therapies for each patient. Some examples of personalized treatment plans using machine learning are:

2.2.1 Depression

Machine learning can help select the best type of psychotherapy (such as cognitive behavioural therapy or psychodynamic therapy) for each depressed patient based on their personality traits, symptoms, and treatment goals [24]. Machine learning can also help predict the treatment outcome and response for each patient based on their baseline characteristics, clinical features, and biomarkers [25].

2.2.2 Cancer

Machine learning can help design personalized vaccines, optimize drug dosages, and select the best therapies for cancer patients based on their genomic profiles, tumour characteristics, and immune system status [26]. Machine learning can also help monitor the treatment efficacy and toxicity for each patient based on their dynamic changes in molecular markers, imaging features, and adverse events [27].

2.2.3 Asthma

Machine learning can help identify the optimal inhaler device, medication regimen, and self-management plan for each asthma patient based on their lung function, inflammation level, environmental exposure, and adherence behaviour. Machine learning can also help detect and prevent asthma exacerbations for each patient based on their real-time symptoms, physiological signals, and environmental triggers.

2.3 Image Analysis and Radiology

Image analysis and radiology represent one of the most promising uses of machine learning in the medical field. Machine learning can help analyse medical images such as X-rays, CT scans, MRI scans, ultrasound images, and microscopy images to detect abnormalities, measure features, segment regions, classify diseases, and predict outcomes. For instance, machine learning can help diagnose breast cancer from mammograms, detect brain tumours from MRI scans, and identify COVID-19 from chest X-rays [28-30]. Machine learning can also assist radiologists in their diagnoses by providing automated annotations, measurements, recommendations, and second opinions [31-34].

Machine learning in image analysis and radiology has the potential to improve the accuracy, efficiency, accessibility, affordability, and safety of healthcare services. However, there are many additional challenges and limitations that need to be addressed, such as data quality, privacy, security, ethics, regulation, interpretability, explainability, trustworthiness, and social impact. Therefore, it is important to develop machine learning methods that are robust, reliable, transparent, fair, accountable, and human-centred for image analysis and radiology applications [35].

2.4 Drug Discovery

Drug discovery is one of the most fascinating uses of machine learning in healthcare. Machine learning can help analyse biological data to identify potential drug candidates and predict their effectiveness. This has the potential to greatly cut down on the time and expense involved in creating new drugs. Some examples of drug discovery using machine learning are [36]:

2.4.1 Molecular Property Prediction

Machine learning can help predict the physicochemical, pharmacokinetic, pharmacodynamic, and toxicological properties of small molecules based on their structures and features. For instance, machine learning can help estimate the solubility, permeability, binding affinity, activity, selectivity, and safety of drug candidates [37-39].

2.4.2. Pretrained Molecular Representations

Machine learning can help learn generalizable and transferable representations of molecules from large-scale unlabelled or labelled data. For example, machine learning can help encode the structural and semantic information of molecules into vectors or graphs that can be used for downstream tasks such as property prediction, similarity search, and de novo design [40].

2.4.3 De novo Molecular Design and Optimization

Machine learning can help generate novel molecules with desired properties and optimize existing molecules to improve their performance. For example, machine learning can help design new antibiotics, antivirals, anticancer agents, and psychedelics using deep generative models, reinforcement learning, and evolutionary algorithms [41].

2.4.4 Retrosynthesis Prediction

Machine learning can help plan the synthesis of target molecules from available starting materials by predicting the optimal sequence of chemical reactions. For instance, machine learning can help automate the synthesis of complex natural products, drugs, and materials using graph neural networks, transformer models, and Monte Carlo tree search [42].

2.4.5. Biomedical Knowledge Graph Reasoning

Machine learning can help infer new knowledge from existing biomedical data by constructing and querying knowledge graphs that represent the entities and relations in the domain. For example, machine learning can help discover new drug-target interactions, drug-disease associations, and drug repurposing opportunities using graph convolutional, and attention networks, and graph embedding methods [43].

Machine learning in drug discovery has the potential to improve the innovation, efficiency, diversity, and quality of healthcare services. However, there are also many challenges and limitations that need to be addressed, such as data quality, privacy, security, ethics, regulation, interpretability, explainability, trustworthiness, and social impact. Therefore, it is important to develop machine learning methods that are robust, reliable, transparent, fair, accountable, and human-centred for drug discovery applications.

3. The Internet of Things in Healthcare

The network of interconnected devices and sensors that collect, transmit, and exchange data over the internet is what is meant by the term Internet of Things. In healthcare, IoT is transforming the way medical devices, patient monitoring, and data management operate. Some examples of the Internet of Things in healthcare are:

3.1 Remote Patient Monitoring (RPM)

IoT enables the continuous and real-time monitoring of patients' vital signs, symptoms, and activities using wearable devices and sensors that are connected to the internet. This allows healthcare providers to remotely access and analyse the patients' data, provide feedback and guidance, and intervene in case of emergencies. RPMs can improve the quality of care, reduce hospitalizations and readmissions, and enhance patient satisfaction and adherence [44]. RPM is a form of telemedicine that uses IoT devices and sensors to collect, transmit, and analyse the health data of patients who are not physically present in a healthcare facility. RPM can provide various benefits for patients and healthcare providers, such as [45]:

3.1.1 Improving the Quality of Care

RPM can enable timely and accurate diagnosis, treatment, and prevention of diseases and health conditions by providing continuous and real-time data on the patients' vital signs, symptoms, and activities. RPM can also facilitate personalized and patient-centred care by allowing the patients to participate in their own health management and receive feedback and guidance from their healthcare providers.

3.1.2 Reducing the Cost of Care

RPM can reduce the need for hospitalizations, readmissions, emergency visits, and transportation costs by allowing the patients to receive care at home or in other convenient locations. RPM can also optimize the use of healthcare resources and personnel by enabling remote consultation, collaboration, and supervision among healthcare providers.

3.1.3 Enhancing the Satisfaction and Adherence of Patients

RPM can improve the convenience, comfort, and accessibility of healthcare services for patients who live in remote areas, have mobility issues, or have busy schedules. RPM can also increase the engagement, motivation, and empowerment of patients by providing them with real-time feedback, reminders, alerts, and incentives.

Some examples of IoT devices and sensors used for RPM are [15]:

- Wearable devices: These are devices that can be worn on the body or attached to clothing or accessories. They can measure various physiological parameters such as heart rate, blood pressure, oxygen saturation, temperature, electrocardiogram (ECG), glucose level, and activity level. They can also provide feedback, alerts, and interventions to the patients and their caregivers. Some examples of wearable devices are smartwatches, fitness trackers, patches, rings, bracelets, necklaces, belts, glasses, earphones, and clothing.
- Non-wearable devices: Non-wearable devices are devices that can be placed in the environment or on other objects. They can measure various environmental parameters such as air quality, humidity, temperature, noise level, light level, and motion. They can also monitor the usage and status of medical equipment such as inhalers, insulin pumps, glucose meters, and medication dispensers. Some examples of non-wearable devices are cameras, microphones, speakers,

smart scales, mirrors, pill bottles, bedsheets, mattresses, pillows, toothbrushes, and toilets.

- Implantable devices: These are devices that can be inserted into the body using surgery or injecting . They can measure various internal parameters such as blood flow, blood pressure, heart rate, electrical activity, temperature, pH level, and oxygen level. They can also deliver drugs, stimulate nerves, or regulate organs [17].

Some examples of implantable devices are pacemakers, defibrillators, neurostimulators, drug pumps, glucose sensors, and biosensors. RPM is a promising technology that can improve the quality, efficiency, accessibility, affordability, and safety of healthcare services.

However, there are also many challenges and limitations that need to be addressed, such as data quality, privacy, security, ethics, regulation, interoperability, scalability, and social impact. Therefore, it is important to develop IoT solutions that are robust, reliable, transparent, fair, accountable, and human-centred for RPM applications.

Figure 4 illustrates the key components and the flow of data in a remote patient monitoring (RPM) scenario that seamlessly integrates smart technology. The aim of this scenario is to enhance the quality and accessibility of healthcare services by leveraging IoT and cloud technologies.

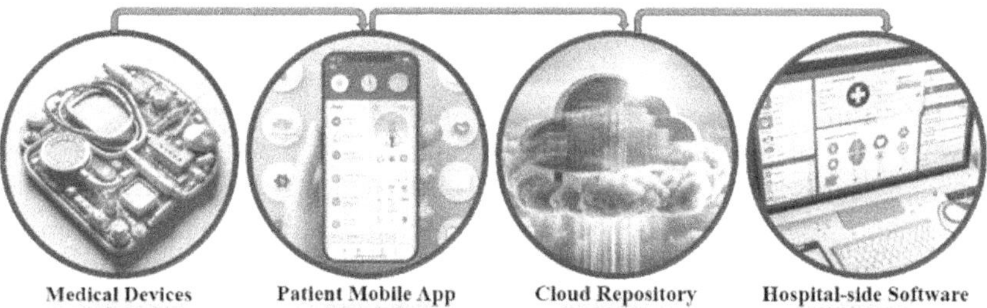

Figure 4. Possible remote patient monitoring scenario using smart phone and IoT cloud

Step 1: Medical Devices

At the beginning of the process, medical devices play a pivotal role. These devices are equipped with sensors that can capture vital health data, such as heart rate, blood pressure, glucose levels, or other relevant parameters. These devices are designed to be user-friendly, enabling patients to easily measure and transmit their health information.

Step 2: Patient Mobile App

The next step involves the patient's active participation. A specialized mobile application, designed for easy installation and use, serves as a bridge between the medical devices and the cloud repository. Patients use the mobile app to connect with the medical devices, collect data, and subsequently transmit it to the cloud.

Step 3: Cloud Repository

This critical stage leverages cloud technology to gather, store, and manage the patient's health data. The cloud repository acts as a centralized hub where information from various patients can be securely stored. This repository can be accessed by healthcare providers, making it an efficient tool for remote patient monitoring.

Step 4: Hospital-Side Software

The final stage of the process is on the healthcare provider's side. They access the cloud repository via dedicated software designed for healthcare professionals. This software allows them to remotely monitor patient data, detect anomalies, and provide timely feedback, advice, or intervention as required. It fosters a patient-provider relationship that transcends the traditional in-person setting.

By connecting medical devices, a user-friendly mobile app, cloud storage, and dedicated healthcare software, this IoT-based scenario opens new avenues for healthcare delivery. It enhances the quality of care by facilitating timely interventions and improving patient engagement, all while reducing the need for frequent in-person hospital visits. However, it's imperative to address challenges related to data quality, privacy, security, ethics, regulation, interoperability, scalability, and social impact when implementing such solutions to ensure they are robust, reliable, and patient-centric.

3.2 Smart Healthcare Facilities

Smart healthcare facilities are those that use IoT sensors and devices to enhance the efficiency and safety of their operations. They can improve the patient experience and reduce the operational costs by implementing the following features [46].

3.2.1 Smart Lighting

Smart lighting systems can adjust the brightness, colour, and temperature of the lights according to the time of day, the occupancy level, the activity level, and the preferences of the patients and staff. They can also save energy by turning off or dimming the lights when they are not needed. Additionally, they can improve the comfort, mood, and sleep quality of the patients and staff [47].

3.2.2 Environmental Monitoring

Environmental monitoring systems can measure and control the temperature, humidity, air quality, noise level, and light level of the indoor environment. They can also detect and alert the presence of harmful substances such as carbon monoxide, smoke, fire, gas, or water leaks. They can also improve the health, safety, and comfort of the patients and staff [48].

3.2.3 Equipment Maintenance

Equipment maintenance systems can monitor and track the status, location, usage, and performance of medical equipment such as ventilators, infusion pumps, monitors, scanners, and defibrillators. They can also notify and schedule the maintenance, repair, or replacement of faulty or outdated equipment and improve the availability, reliability, and quality of medical equipment [49].

Smart healthcare facilities are a promising technology that can improve the quality, efficiency, accessibility, affordability, and safety of healthcare services. However, a number of issues and constraints must also be resolved, including those pertaining to data quality, privacy, security, ethics, regulation, interoperability, scalability, and societal impact. Therefore, it is important to develop IoT solutions that are robust, reliable, transparent, fair, accountable, and human-centred for smart healthcare facilities applications.

3.3 Medication Management

Medication management is the process of ensuring that patients take their medications as prescribed, and that they are safe, effective, and appropriate for their conditions. Medication errors, adverse drug events, drug interactions, and non-adherence can all be avoided with medication management, which can lower health outcomes and raise healthcare expenses. IoT devices and systems can help improve medication management by providing the following features:

3.3.1 Smart Pill Dispensers

Smart pill dispensers are devices that store, organize, and dispense medications for patients. They can remind the patients when to take their medications, provide the correct dosage and instructions, and lock the medications until the scheduled time. They can also alert the patients and their caregivers if they miss a dose, take a wrong dose, or run out of medication. Some examples of smart pill dispensers are MedMinder, Philips Medication Dispensing Service, and Hero [50].

3.3.2 Medication Adherence Monitoring Systems

Medication adherence monitoring systems are devices or apps that track and record the medication usage of patients. They can use various methods such as barcode scanning, pill bottle opening, weight sensing, or biometric sensing to verify that the patients have taken their medications. They can also provide feedback, incentives, or interventions to improve the adherence of the patients. Some examples of medication adherence monitoring systems are Proteus Digital Health, Medisafe, and AiCure [51].

IoT devices and systems can help improve medication management by providing convenience, accuracy, and accountability for patients and healthcare providers. However, there are also many challenges and limitations that need to be addressed, such as data quality, privacy, security, ethics, regulation, interoperability, scalability, and social impact. Therefore, it is important to develop IoT solutions that are robust, reliable, transparent, fair, accountable, and human-centered for medication management applications.

4. Synergies between Machine Learning and IoT in Healthcare

The true power of ML and IoT in healthcare emerges when these technologies are combined. IoT devices generate vast amounts of real-time data, which ML algorithms can analyze to provide actionable insights. For example:

4.1 Early Warning Systems (EWS)

EWS are those that use IoT sensors and ML models to detect and alert the occurrence or risk of adverse events, such as cardiac arrest, sepsis, or falls, in hospital settings. EWS can improve patient safety, quality of care, and clinical outcomes by enabling timely and appropriate interventions [52]. Some examples of EWS using ML and IoT are:

4.1.1 The e-Alert System

The e-Alert system is an EWS that uses IoT sensors to monitor patients' vital signs, such as heart rate, blood pressure, respiratory rate, and oxygen saturation, and transmit them to a cloud-based ML model. The ML model analyses the data and calculates a risk score for each patient based on their condition and history. The risk score is then displayed on a dashboard and sent to the clinicians' smartphones or tablets. The e-Alert system can help identify patients who are at risk of deterioration or cardiac arrest and alert the rapid response team for timely intervention [53].

4.1.2 The Sepsis Watch System

The Sepsis Watch system is an EWS that uses IoT devices to collect patients' electronic health records (EHRs), laboratory results, and vital signs, and feed them to a cloud-based ML model. The ML model uses a deep learning approach to predict the probability of sepsis onset for each patient based on their data. The probability is then displayed on a dashboard and sent to the clinicians' smartphones or tablets. The Sepsis Watch system can help diagnose sepsis early and initiate appropriate treatment protocols [16, 54, 55].

4.1.3 The Foresight System

The Foresight system is an EWS that uses IoT sensors to monitor patients' movements, posture, gait, and activity level, and send them to a cloud-based ML model. The ML model uses a machine vision approach to detect abnormal patterns or behaviours that may indicate a fall risk for each patient. The risk level is then displayed on a dashboard and sent to the clinicians' smartphones or tablets. The Foresight system can help prevent falls and injuries by providing feedback, guidance, and alerts to the patients and staff [56].

EWS using ML and IoT have the potential to improve the accuracy, efficiency, accessibility, affordability, and safety of healthcare services. However, a number of issues and constraints must also be resolved, including those pertaining to data quality, privacy, security, ethics, regulation, interoperability, scalability, and societal impact. Therefore, it is important to develop EWS solutions that are robust, reliable, transparent, fair, accountable, and human-centred for healthcare applications.

4.2 Predictive Maintenance

IoT sensors and machine learning algorithms are used in predictive maintenance (PdM), a proactive strategy to maintain the best possible performance and dependability of medical equipment by predicting when repair is necessary. PdM can help reduce the downtime, cost, and risk associated with equipment failure, breakdown, or malfunction [56]. Some examples of PdM using ML and IoT are:

4.2.1 The Smart Hospital System

The Smart Hospital system is a PdM system that uses IoT sensors to collect data from various medical equipments such as ventilators, infusion pumps, monitors, scanners, and defibrillators. The data is then sent to a cloud-based ML model that analyses the data and predicts the remaining useful life, health status, and failure probability of each equipment. The predictions are then displayed on a dashboard and sent to the maintenance staff's smartphones or tablets. The Smart Hospital system can help schedule and prioritize the maintenance tasks based on the urgency and importance of each equipment [57].

4.2.2 The Prognosis System

The Prognosis system is a PdM system that uses IoT devices to collect data from implantable medical devices such as pacemakers, defibrillators, neurostimulators, and drug pumps. The data is then sent to a cloud-based ML model that analyzes the data and predicts the battery life, device performance, and patient outcome of each device. The predictions are then displayed on a dashboard and sent to the clinicians' smartphones or tablets. The Prognosis system can help optimize the device settings, plan the device replacement, and monitor the patient condition [58].

4.2.3 The MedSense System

The MedSense system is a PdM system that uses IoT sensors to collect data from non-invasive medical devices such as glucose meters, blood pressure monitors, thermometers, and pulse oximeters. The data is then sent to a cloud-based ML model that analyzes the data and predicts the calibration and measurement errors. Additionally, it analyses any device malfunction . The predictions are then displayed on a dashboard and sent to the users' smartphones or tablets. The MedSense system can help ensure the accuracy, quality, and reliability of the device measurements [59].

PdM using ML and IoT have the potential to improve the quality, efficiency, accessibility, affordability, and safety of healthcare services. However, there are also many challenges and limitations that need to be addressed, such as data quality, privacy, security, ethics, regulation, interoperability, scalability, and social impact. Therefore, it is important to develop PdM solutions that are robust, reliable, transparent, fair, accountable, and human-centred for healthcare applications.

4.3 Patient-Centred Care

Patient-centered care (PCC) is a care approach that respects and responds to the individual needs, preferences, and values of each patient in all clinical decisions [60]. PCC can improve the quality, effectiveness, and satisfaction of healthcare services by involving the patient as an equal partner in the design and delivery of care [61]. By analysing data from wearable IoT devices, ML can provide healthcare providers with a comprehensive view of a patient's health and behaviour (Figure 5). This holistic approach enables more personalized and effective care plans. Some examples of PCC using ML and IoT are:

4.3.1 The CareMore System

The CareMore system is a PCC system that uses IoT devices such as smartwatches, fitness trackers, and blood pressure monitors to collect data from patients with chronic conditions such as diabetes, hypertension, and heart failure. The data is then sent to a cloud-based ML model that analyzes the data and provides personalized feedback, recommendations, and interventions to the patients and their care teams. The CareMore system can help improve the self-management, adherence, and patient outcomes [62].

4.3.2 The iCare System

The iCare system is a PCC system that uses IoT devices such as smart glasses, gloves, and shoes to collect data from patients with dementia or Alzheimer's disease. The data is then sent to a cloud-based ML model that analyzes the data and provides personalized reminders, prompts, and assistance to the patients and their caregivers. The iCare system can help improve the cognitive function, independence, and patients' quality of life.

4.3.3 The Wellframe System

The Wellframe system is a PCC system that uses IoT devices such as smartphones, tablets, and smart speakers to collect data from patients with various health conditions such as depression, anxiety, asthma, and chronic pain. The data is then sent to a cloud-based ML model that analyzes the data and provides personalized content, coaching, and support to the patients and their healthcare providers. The Wellframe system can help improve engagement, motivation, and patients' recovery [63].

PCC using ML and IoT have the potential to improve the quality, efficiency, accessibility, affordability, and healthcare services' safety . However, there are also many challenges and limitations that need to be addressed, such as data quality, privacy, security, ethics, regulation, interoperability, scalability, and social impact. Therefore, it is important to develop PCC solutions that are robust, reliable, transparent, fair, accountable and human-centred for healthcare applications.

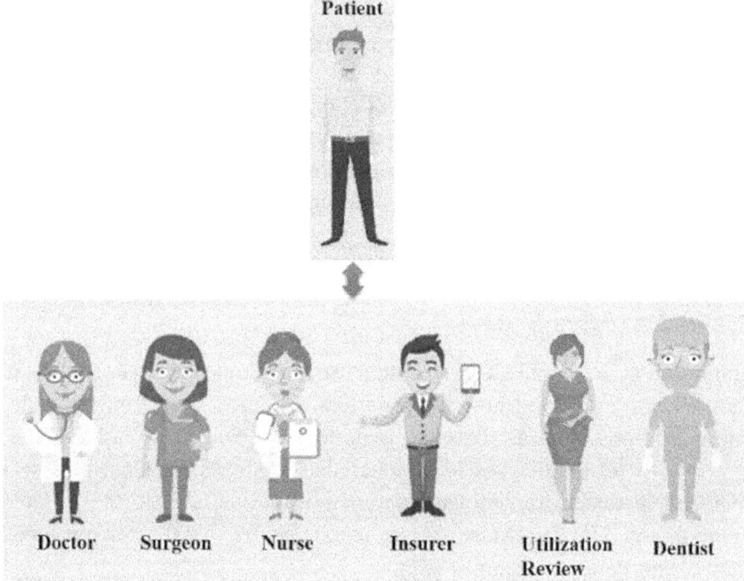

Figure 5. Patient centric maintenance

5. Challenges and Considerations

While ML and IoT offer tremendous promise in healthcare. Several challenges and considerations must be addressed to ensure their ethical, legal, and social implications and appropriate handling. In this section, we will discuss some of the major challenges and considerations that healthcare organizations and stakeholders should be aware of and address them when implementing ML and IoT solutions in healthcare.

5.1 Data Privacy and Security

One of the most critical challenges and considerations for ML and IoT in healthcare is data privacy and security. To maintain patient privacy and adhere to regulations such as the Health Insurance Portability and Accountability Act (HIPAA), a significant quantity of sensitive healthcare data, including location, genetic, biometric, and personal health information, generated by Internet of Things (IoT) devices, needs to be protected [64]. Data privacy and security involve ensuring that data is collected, stored, transmitted, processed, and shared in a secure and confidential manner, with the consent of the data subjects or their authorized representatives, and for authorized objectives only [65]. Data privacy and security also involve preventing unauthorized access, use, disclosure, modification, or destruction of data by malicious actors or accidental errors [66].

Data privacy and security are challenging for ML and IoT in healthcare for several reasons. First, the large volume, variety, velocity, and veracity of data generated by IoT devices pose technical challenges for data encryption, authentication, authorization, backup, recovery, and auditing [67]. Second, the distributed and heterogeneous nature of IoT devices and networks pose architectural challenges for data governance, standardization, interoperability, and compliance [68]. Third, the dynamic and complex nature of ML algorithms pose analytical challenges for data quality, validity, reliability, transparency, explainability, and accountability. Fourth, the diverse and evolving nature of data stakeholders pose ethical challenges for data ownership, control, access, sharing, benefit, harm, and responsibility [69].

Data privacy and security are essential for ML and IoT in healthcare to ensure the trust, confidence, and participation of patients and other stakeholders. Data privacy and security also have legal implications for healthcare organizations as they may face penalties or lawsuits if they fail to comply with the relevant regulations or standards. Consequently, the following actions should be part of healthcare organizations' comprehensive and proactive approaches to data privacy and security [70]:

- Conduct a risk assessment to identify the potential threats and vulnerabilities to data privacy and security in ML and IoT applications.
- Implement appropriate technical measures to protect data at rest, in transit or in use. These may include encryption, hashing, anonymization, pseudonymization, firewalls, antivirus software, and intrusion detection systems [71, 72].
- Implement appropriate organizational measures to manage data governance, policies, procedures, roles, and responsibilities. These may include data protection officers, data stewards, data quality assurance teams, and data breach response teams.
- Implement appropriate legal measures to comply with the applicable regulations, standards, and contracts. These may include consent forms, privacy notices, data sharing agreements, and data protection impact assessments.
- Implement appropriate ethical measures to respect the rights, interests, and

values of data subjects and other stakeholders. These may include ethical principles, codes of conduct, and ethical review boards.

5.2 Data Quality and Standardization

Data quality and standardization are important challenges and considerations for ML and IoT in healthcare. Data quality refers to the degree to which data meets the expectations and requirements of the data consumers, such as accuracy, completeness, consistency, timeliness, and validity [73]. The act of converting data into a uniform format and structure that complies with established guidelines, including name, coding, classification, and representation, is known as data standardization [74]. Data quality and standardization are essential for ensuring the accuracy and reliability of ML models, as well as the interoperability and integration of IoT devices and systems [75].

Data quality and standardization are challenging for ML and IoT in healthcare for several reasons. First, the large volume, variety, velocity, and veracity of data generated by IoT devices pose technical challenges for data collection, validation, cleaning, integration, and labelling [76]. Second, the distributed and heterogeneous nature of IoT devices and networks pose architectural challenges for data governance, coordination, synchronization, and alignment. Third, the dynamic and complex nature of ML algorithms pose analytical challenges for data evaluation, interpretation, explanation, and feedback [74]. Fourth, the diverse and evolving nature of data stakeholders pose ethical challenges for data ownership, control, access, sharing, benefit, harm, and responsibility.

Data quality and standardization are important for improving the quality, efficiency, accessibility, affordability, and safety of healthcare services. Data quality and standardization also have legal implications for healthcare organizations as they may face penalties or lawsuits if they fail to comply with the relevant regulations or standards. Therefore, healthcare organizations should adopt a comprehensive and proactive approach to data quality and standardization that involves the following steps:

- Conduct a data quality assessment to identify the current state of data quality in terms of dimensions, metrics, sources, causes, and impacts of data quality issues.
- Implement appropriate data quality improvement methods to address the identified data quality issues. These may include data cleansing, deduplication, normalization, enrichment, and verification.
- Implement appropriate data standardization methods to transform data into a common format and structure. These may include data element naming standards [76], data classification standards, data representation standards [74], and data exchange standards.
- Implement appropriate data quality monitoring methods to measure and track the changes in data quality over time. These may include data quality dashboards, reports, and alerts.

- Implement appropriate data quality management methods to ensure the sustainability of data quality practices. These may include data quality policies, procedures, roles, and responsibilities.

5.3 Integration and Interoperability

Integration and interoperability are key challenges and considerations for ML and IoT in healthcare. Integration refers to the process of combining IoT devices and ML systems with existing healthcare infrastructure, such as electronic health records (EHRs), clinical decision support systems (CDSSs), and health information exchanges (HIEs). Interoperability refers to the ability of IoT devices and ML systems to communicate and exchange data with each other and with other healthcare systems, using common standards, protocols, and interfaces. Integration and interoperability are essential for realizing the full potential of ML and IoT in healthcare, as they can enable the following benefits:

5.3.1 Improved Quality of Care

Integration and interoperability can improve the quality of care by providing a comprehensive and holistic view of the patient's health status, history, and needs, as well as the available resources, services, and interventions. This can facilitate accurate diagnosis, effective treatment, and personalized care plans for each patient.

5.3.2 Reduced cost of care

Integration and interoperability can reduce the cost of care by eliminating data silos, redundancies, errors, and delays that result from incompatible or isolated systems. This can optimize the use of healthcare resources, personnel, and equipment, as well as reduce unnecessary tests, procedures, or hospitalizations.

5.3.3 Enhanced Patient Satisfaction

Integration and interoperability can enhance patient satisfaction by providing convenience, accessibility, transparency, and empowerment to the patients. This can enable the patients to access their own health data, receive feedback and guidance from their healthcare providers, participate in their own care management, and share their data with other stakeholders.

Integration and interoperability are challenging for ML and IoT in healthcare for several reasons. First, the large volume, variety, velocity, and veracity of data generated by IoT devices pose technical challenges for data integration, aggregation, transformation, and analysis. Second, the distributed and heterogeneous nature of IoT devices and networks pose architectural challenges for data coordination, synchronization, alignment, and governance. Third, the dynamic and complex nature of ML algorithms pose analytical challenges for data evaluation, interpretation, explanation, and feedback. Fourth, the diverse and evolving nature of data stakeholders pose ethical challenges for data ownership, control, access, sharing, benefit, harm, and responsibility.

Integration and interoperability are important for improving the quality, efficiency, accessibility, affordability, and safety of healthcare services. Integration and interoperability also have legal implications for healthcare organizations as they may face penalties or lawsuits if they fail to comply with the relevant regulations or standards. Therefore, healthcare organizations should adopt a comprehensive and proactive approach to integration and interoperability that involves the following steps:

- Conduct a gap analysis to identify the current state of integration and interoperability in terms of capabilities, requirements, and challenges.
- Implement appropriate integration methods to connect IoT devices and ML systems with existing healthcare infrastructure. These may include application programming interfaces (APIs), middleware platforms, and cloud computing services.
- Implement appropriate interoperability methods to enable data communication and exchange among IoT devices and ML systems and with other healthcare systems. These may include data standards, protocols, and interfaces.
- Implement appropriate integration monitoring methods to measure and track the performance and impact of integration and interoperability on healthcare outcomes. These may include integration dashboards, reports, and alerts.
- Implement appropriate integration management methods to ensure the sustainability of integration and interoperability practices. These may include integration policies, procedures, roles, and responsibilities.

5.4 Ethical and Regulatory Challenges

As AI and IoT applications in healthcare grow, ethical and regulatory challenges must be carefully considered to ensure the respect, dignity, and rights of the patients and other stakeholders. Ethical and regulatory challenges involve addressing the moral, legal, and social implications of using ML and IoT in healthcare, such as algorithmic bias, accountability, transparency, consent, privacy, security, safety, quality, and trust [70]. Ethical and regulatory challenges are important for ensuring the fairness, justice, and responsibility of ML and IoT in healthcare, as well as the compliance with the relevant laws, standards, and guidelines.

Ethical and regulatory challenges are challenging for ML and IoT in healthcare for several reasons. First, the large volume, variety, velocity, and veracity of data generated by IoT devices pose ethical challenges for data ownership, control, access, sharing, benefit, harm, and responsibility [77]. Second, the distributed and heterogeneous nature of IoT devices and networks pose ethical challenges for data governance, coordination, synchronization, alignment, and governance [78]. Third, the dynamic and complex nature of ML algorithms pose ethical challenges for data quality, validity, reliability, transparency, explainability, and accountability. Fourth, the diverse and evolving nature of data stakeholders pose ethical challenges for data consent, privacy, security, safety, quality, and trust [78].

Ethical and regulatory challenges are important for improving the quality, efficiency, accessibility, affordability, and safety of healthcare services. Ethical and regulatory challenges also have legal implications for healthcare organizations as they may face penalties or lawsuits if they fail to comply with the relevant regulations or standards. Therefore, healthcare organizations should adopt a comprehensive and proactive approach to ethical and regulatory challenges that involves the following steps:

- Conduct an ethical and regulatory assessment to identify the potential risks and benefits of using ML and IoT in healthcare for the patients and other stakeholders.
- Implement appropriate ethical and regulatory measures to mitigate the risks and maximize the benefits of using ML and IoT in healthcare. These may include ethical principles, codes of conduct, and ethical review boards.
- Implement appropriate ethical and regulatory monitoring methods to measure and track the impact and outcomes of using ML and IoT in healthcare. These may include ethical and regulatory dashboards, reports, and alerts.
- Implement appropriate ethical and regulatory management methods to ensure the sustainability of ethical and regulatory practices. These may include ethical and regulatory policies, procedures, roles, and responsibilities.

6. Future Directions

The integration of Machine Learning and the Internet of Things in healthcare is an ongoing journey with limitless possibilities. Future directions may include:

6.1 AI-Powered Virtual Health Assistants

AI-driven virtual assistants are applications that use natural language processing and generation to interact with patients through voice or text, providing them with real-time health advice and reminders, improving self-management and adherence to treatment plans [79]. These assistants can also collect and analyze data from various sources, such as electronic health records, wearable devices, sensors, and online platforms, to provide personalized and context-aware information and guidance. AI-powered virtual assistants can potentially improve the quality of care by enhancing patient engagement, satisfaction, education, and empowerment, as well as reducing the burden on healthcare professionals and systems [80]. Some examples of AI-powered virtual assistants in healthcare are:

6.1.1 Ada

A chatbot that helps users to assess their symptoms, understand their health conditions, and find appropriate care options [81].

6.1.2 Babylon

A virtual health service that provides users with access to online consultations, health assessments, prescriptions, referrals, and health records [82].

6.1.3 Woebot

A chatbot that delivers cognitive behavioural therapy for users with mental health issues, such as depression and anxiety [83].

6.1.4 Molly

A chatbot that acts as a personal health assistant for chronic disease management, providing users with medication reminders, health tips, and motivational messages. However, with the rapid advancement of AI and IoT technologies, as well as the increasing demand for convenient and accessible healthcare services, AI-powered virtual assistants are expected to play a more prominent role in the future of healthcare [84].

AI-powered virtual assistants are still in their early stages of development and implementation, and face several challenges and limitations, such as data privacy and security, user trust and acceptance, technical reliability and accuracy, ethical and regulatory issues, and integration and interoperability with existing healthcare systems.

6.2 Population Health Management (PHM)

Population health management (PHM) is a proactive approach to enhance the health and well-being of a targeted population by addressing health determinants, reducing health disparities, and optimizing health outcomes and costs through the use of data, analytics, and interventions [85]. ML and IoT can help healthcare systems implement PHM by providing the following capabilities [86]:

6.2.1 Data Integration and Aggregation

In order to create a thorough and comprehensive picture of the population's health status, needs, and risks, healthcare systems can benefit from the use of ML and IoT to gather and integrate "data from various sources, such as electronic health records, wearable devices," sensors, social media, and environmental factors [87].

6.2.2 Data Analysis and Segmentation

ML and IoT can help healthcare systems analyse and segment data using advanced techniques, such as clustering, classification, regression, and natural language processing, to identify patterns, trends, gaps, and opportunities for improving population health [88-91].

6.2.3 Data Visualization and Dissemination

ML and IoT can help healthcare systems visualize and disseminate data using interactive dashboards, reports, and alerts, to provide actionable insights and feedback to the stakeholders involved in PHM, such as clinicians, managers, policymakers, and patients [85].

6.2.4 Data-Driven Intervention Design and Evaluation

ML and IoT can help healthcare systems design and evaluate interventions based on data-driven evidence, such as predictive modelling, causal inference, optimization, and reinforcement learning, to provide personalized and preventive care for the population [86].

ML and IoT can potentially improve the quality, efficiency, accessibility, affordability, and safety of healthcare services by enabling PHM. However, a number of issues and constraints must also be resolved, including those pertaining to data quality, privacy, security, ethics, regulation, interoperability, scalability, and societal impact. Therefore, it is important to develop ML and IoT solutions that are robust, reliable, transparent, fair, accountable, and human-centred for PHM applications.

6.3 Drug Personalization

Drug personalization is the process of designing and delivering drugs that are tailored to an individual's genetics and health profile, such as their disease, symptoms, biomarkers, metabolism, and response to treatment. Drug personalization can potentially improve the efficacy and safety of drugs by reducing adverse effects, increasing therapeutic effects, and optimizing dosing regimens [92]. AI and IoT can enable drug personalization by providing the following capabilities [93]:

6.3.1 Data Generation and Collection

AI and IoT can help generate and collect data from various sources, such as genomic sequencing, transcriptomic profiling, proteomic analysis, metabolomic measurement, microbiome assessment, and phenotypic observation, to create a comprehensive and dynamic view of the individual's molecular and clinical characteristics [94, 95].

6.3.2 Data Integration and Analysis

AI and IoT can help integrate and analyse data using advanced techniques, such as machine learning, deep learning, network analysis, and systems biology, to identify the molecular mechanisms, pathways, targets, and biomarkers involved in the individual's disease and drug response [96].

6.3.3 Data-driven Drug Design and Delivery

AI and IoT can help design and deliver drugs based on data-driven evidence, such as molecular docking, virtual screening, structure-based drug design, pharmacophore modelling, drug repurposing, nanotechnology, smart devices, and digital therapeutics.

AI and IoT can potentially revolutionize the field of drug personalization by enabling the development of truly personalized medications that are customized to each individual's unique genetic and health profile. However, there are also many challenges and limitations that need to be addressed, such as data quality, privacy, security, ethics, regulation, interoperability, scalability, and social impact. Therefore, it is important to develop AI and IoT solutions that are robust, reliable, transparent, fair, accountable, and human-centred for drug personalization applications.

7. Conclusion

In conclusion, the integration of Machine Learning (ML) and the Internet of Things (IoT) in healthcare represents a transformative development with tremendous potential for the future of medicine. Throughout this chapter, we have explored the multifaceted landscape of ML and IoT applications in healthcare, witnessing their profound impact on how we approach, deliver, and experience medical care. From real-time monitoring of vital signs to the early detection of adverse events through Early Warning Systems (EWS), ML and IoT have already begun to revolutionize patient care within hospital settings. Predictive Maintenance (PdM) offers the promise of reducing equipment downtime and ensuring the optimal performance of medical devices, while Patient-Centered Care (PCC) paves the way for more personalized and engaging healthcare experiences. However, these groundbreaking advancements do not come without their set of challenges and considerations. Data privacy and security are of paramount concern, as healthcare organizations grapple with safeguarding sensitive patient data while complying with rigorous regulations. Data quality and standardization remain pivotal in ensuring the accuracy and reliability of ML models, and the need for integration and interoperability remains essential for seamless healthcare delivery. Ethical and regulatory considerations serve as guiding principles in navigating the complex landscape of AI and IoT applications in healthcare. Ensuring fairness, transparency, and accountability in the development and deployment of these technologies is crucial to maintaining public trust and adhering to legal obligations.

Looking ahead, the future of ML and IoT in healthcare holds exciting possibilities. AI-powered virtual health assistants, poised to offer real-time guidance and support to patients, have the potential to enhance engagement and reduce the burden on healthcare professionals. Population Health Management (PHM) promises to create a more holistic and data-driven approach to healthcare, while drug personalization offers the tantalizing prospect of tailored treatments based on individual genetic and health profiles. As we move forward into the future, it is imperative that we remain vigilant, addressing the challenges and ethical considerations that arise along the way. By doing so, we can harness the full potential of ML and IoT in healthcare, ultimately advancing the quality, accessibility, and safety of medical services for all. In the ever-evolving realm of healthcare technology, ML and IoT stand as powerful allies, offering innovative solutions to age-old challenges. With careful planning, ethical diligence, and a commitment to patient-centric care, the integration of ML and IoT is poised to lead us toward a brighter, more efficient, and healthier future in healthcare.

References

[1] Shariaty, F. and Mousavi, M. Application of CAD systems for the automatic detection of lung nodules. Informatics in Medicine Unlocked, 15: 100173, 2019.

[2] Shariaty, F., Baranov, M. and Tsybin, O. Automatization of biofilms image processing for biomolecular electronics and life science. *In:* 2022 International Conference on Electrical Engineering and Photonics (EExPolytech). 2022. IEEE.

[3] Faridoddin, S. Identification of signs of human lung damage by computer methods: Final qualifying work of the master: direction 11.04. 02 "Infocommunication technologies and communication systems"; educational program 11.04. 02_07 "Laser and fiber optic systems (international educational program)". 2021.

[4] Roy, S.S., Pratyush, C. and Barna, C. Predicting ozone layer concentration using multivariate adaptive regression splines, random forest and classification and regression tree. *In:* Soft Computing Applications: Proceedings of the 7th International Workshop Soft Computing Applications (SOFA 2016), Volume 2 7. 2018. Springer.

[5] Shariaty, F., Shariati, S., Navvabi, S., Oshnari, M.N. and Novikov, B. Application of Artificial Intelligence for Rapid Prevention of Epidemic Diseases (COVID-19). 2022.

[6] Butt, U.M., Letchmunan, S., Ali, M., Hassan, F.H., Baqir, A. and Sherazi, H.H.R. Machine learning based diabetes classification and prediction for healthcare applications. Journal of Healthcare Engineering, 2021.

[7] Ravaut, M., Harish, V., Sadeghi, H., Leung, K.K., Volkovs, M., Kornas, K. et al. Development and validation of a machine learning model using administrative health data to predict onset of type 2 diabetes. JAMA Network Open, 4(5): e2111315-e2111315, 2021.

[8] Zou, Q., Qu, K., Luo, Y., Yin, D., Ju, Y. and Tang, H. Predicting diabetes mellitus with machine learning techniques. Frontiers in Genetics, 9: 515, 2018.

[9] El_Jerjawi, N.S. and Abu-Naser, S.S. Diabetes Prediction Using Artificial Neural Network. 2018.

[10] Shariaty, F., Baranov, M., Velichko, E., Galeeva, M. and Pavlov V. Radiomics: Extracting more features using endoscopic imaging. *In:* 2019 IEEE International Conference on Electrical Engineering and Photonics (EExPolytech). 2019. IEEE.

[11] Roy, S.S., Viswanatham, V.M., Krishna, P.V., Saraf, N., Gupta, A. and Mishra, R. Applicability of rough set technique for data investigation and optimization of intrusion detection system. *In:* Quality, Reliability, Security and Robustness in Heterogeneous Networks: 9th International Conference, QShine 2013, Greater

Noida, India, January 11-12, 2013, Revised Selected Papers 9. 2013. Springer.
[12] Alfayez, A.A., Kunz, H. and Lai, A.G. Predicting the risk of cancer in adults using supervised machine learning: A scoping review. BMJ Open, 11(9): e047755, 2021.
[13] Ebrahimi, M., Novikov, B., Ebrahimie, E., Spilman, A., Ahsan, R., Tahsili, M.R. et al. The first report of the most important sequential differences between COVID-19 and MERS viruses by attribute weighting models, the importance of Nucleocapsid (N) protein. 2020.
[14] Mohammad, R., Nader, M., Faridoddin, S. and Aleksandr, G. Potential of brain-computer interfaces in dementia. *In:* 2023 International Conference on Electrical Engineering and Photonics (EExPolytech). 2023. IEEE.
[15] Mohammed, K., Zaidan, A., Zaidan, B., Albahri, O.S., Alsalem, M., Albahri, A.S. et al. Real-time remote-health monitoring systems: A review on patients prioritisation for multiple-chronic diseases, taxonomy analysis, concerns and solution procedure. Journal of Medical Systems, 43: 1-21, 2019.
[16] Roy, S.S., Gupta, A., Sinha, A. and Ramesh R. Cancer data investigation using variable precision rough set with flexible classification. *In:* Proceedings of the Second International Conference on Computational Science, Engineering and Information Technology. 2012.
[17] Roy, S.S. and Taguchi, Y.-H. Identification of genes associated with altered gene expression and m6A profiles during hypoxia using tensor decomposition based unsupervised feature extraction. Scientific Reports, 11(1): 8909, 2021.
[18] Samui, P., Kim, D., Jagan, J. and Roy, S.S. Determination of uplift capacity of suction caisson using Gaussian process regression, minimax probability machine regression and extreme learning machine. Iranian Journal of Science and Technology, Transactions of Civil Engineering, 43: 651-657, 2019.
[19] Velichko, E., Shariaty, F., Orooji, M., Pavlov, V., Pervunina. T., Zavjalov, S. et al. Development of computer-aided model to differentiate COVID-19 from pulmonary edema in lung CT scan: EDECOVID-net. Computers in Biology and Medicine, 141: 105172, 2022.
[20] Pavlov, V.A., Shariaty, F., Orooji, M. and Velichko, E.N. Application of deep learning techniques for detection of COVID-19 using lung CT scans: Model development and validation. *In:* International Youth Conference on Electronics, Telecommunications and Information Technologies: Proceedings of the YETI 2021, St. Petersburg, Russia. 2022. Springer.
[21] Shariaty, F., Pavlov, V., Velichko, E., Pervunina, T. and Orooji, M. Severity and progression quantification of Covid-19 in CT images: A new deep-learning approach. *In:* 2021 International Conference on Electrical Engineering and Photonics (EExPolytech). 2021. IEEE.
[22] Shariaty, F., Pavlov, V.A., Zavyalov, S., Orooji, M. and Pervunina, T.M. Application of a texture appearance model for segmentation of lung nodules on computed tomography of the chest. Journal of the Russian Universities, 25(3): 97, 1998.
[23] Shariaty, F., Orooji, M., Velichko, E.N. and Zavjalov, S.V. Texture appearance model, a new model-based segmentation paradigm, application on the segmentation of lung nodule in the CT scan of the chest. Computers in Biology and Medicine, 140: 105086, 2022.
[24] Schwartz, B., Cohen, Z.D., Rubel, J.A., Zimmermann, D., Wittmann, W.W. and Lutz, W. Personalized treatment selection in routine care: Integrating machine learning

and statistical algorithms to recommend cognitive behavioral or psychodynamic therapy. Psychotherapy Research, 31(1): 33-51, 2021.

[25] Webb, C.A., Cohen, Z.D., Beard, C., Forgeard, M., Peckham, A.D. and Björgvinsson, T. Personalized prognostic prediction of treatment outcome for depressed patients in a naturalistic psychiatric hospital setting: A comparison of machine learning approaches. Journal of Consulting and Clinical Psychology, 88(1): 25, 2020.

[26] Peng, J., Jury, E.C., Dönnes, P. and Ciurtin, C. Machine learning techniques for personalised medicine approaches in immune-mediated chronic inflammatory diseases: Applications and challenges. Frontiers in Pharmacology, 12: 720694, 2021.

[27] Deng, J., Hartung, T., Capobianco, E., Chen, J.Y. and Emmert-Streib, F. Artificial intelligence for precision medicine. Frontiers in Artificial Intelligence, 4: 834645, 2022.

[28] Montagnon, E., Cerny, M., Cadrin-Chênevert, A., Hamilton, V., Derennes, T., Ilinca, A. et al. Deep learning workflow in radiology: A primer. Insights into Imaging, 11: 1-15, 2020.

[29] Ghoshal, N., Anas, M. and Roy, S.S. Chest X-ray image classification of pneumonia disease using EfficientNet and InceptionV3. Deep Learning Applications in Image Analysis, pp. 173-186, 2023. Springer.

[30] Faridoddin, S. and O. Mahdi, Inf-Seg: Automatic segmentation and quantification method for CT-based COVID-19 diagnosis. Computer Science, Telecommunications and Management, 15(3): 7-21, 2022.

[31] Wang, S., Cao, G., Wang, Y., Liao, S., Wang, Q., Shi, J. et al. Review and prospect: Artificial intelligence in advanced medical imaging. Frontiers in Radiology, 1: 781868, 2021.

[32] Shariaty, F., Duan, L., Pavlov, V., Mousavi, M. and Pervunina, T. A novel gene assay combined with medical imaging for accurate prognosis and prediction of cancer type. *In:* 2022 International Conference on Electrical Engineering and Photonics (EExPolytech). 2022. IEEE.

[33] Nayak, S.R., Nayak, D.R., Sinha, U., Arora, V. and Pachori, R.B. Application of deep learning techniques for detection of COVID-19 cases using chest X-ray images: A comprehensive study. Biomedical Signal Processing and Control, 64: 102365, 2021.

[34] Shariaty, F., Hosseinlou, S. and Rud, V.Y. Automatic lung segmentation method in computed tomography scans. *In:* Journal of Physics: Conference Series. 2019. IOP Publishing.

[35] Shariaty, F., Mousavi, M., Moradi, A., Oshnari, M.N., Navvabi, S., Orooji, M. et al. Semi-automatic segmentation of COVID-19 infection in lung CT scans. *In:* International Youth Conference on Electronics, Telecommunications and Information Technologies: Proceedings of the YETI 2021, St. Petersburg, Russia. 2022. Springer.

[36] Faridoddin, S., Maksim, B. and Oleg, T. Quantitative analysis of biomolecular films: Automated detection and characterization of leaves and spiral structures. *In:* 2023 International Conference on Electrical Engineering and Photonics (EExPolytech). 2023. IEEE.

[37] Dara, S., Dhamercherla, S., Jadav, S.S., Babu, C.M. and Ahsan, M.J. Machine learning in drug discovery: A review. Artificial Intelligence Review, 55(3): 1947-1999, 2022.

[38] Maria, S., Faridoddin, S., Sergey, R. and Amir Reza, R. Personalized chemotherapy selection for lung cancer patients using machine learning and computed tomography.

In: 2023 International Conference on Electrical Engineering and Photonics (EExPolytech). 2023. IEEE.

[39] Baranov, M., Velichko, E. and Shariaty, F. Determination of geometrical parameters in blood serum films using an image segmentation algorithm. Optical Memory and Neural Networks, 29: 330-335, 2020.

[40] Zhu, Z., Shi, C., Zhang, Z., Liu, S., Xu, M., Yuan, X. et al. Torchdrug: A powerful and flexible machine learning platform for drug discovery. arXiv preprint arXiv:2202.08320, 2022.

[41] Gaudelet, T., Day, B., Jamasb, A.R., Soman, J., Regep, C., Liu, G. et al. Utilizing graph machine learning within drug discovery and development. Briefings in Bioinformatics, 22(6): bbab159, 2021.

[42] Li, J., Alam, M., Congzhou, M.S., Wang, J., Dokholyan, N.V. and Ghosh, S. Drug discovery approaches using quantum machine learning. *In:* 2021 58th ACM/IEEE Design Automation Conference (DAC). 2021. IEEE.

[43] Hu, W., Liu, Y., Chen, X., Chai, W., Chen, H., Wang, H. et al. Deep learning methods for small molecule drug discovery: A survey. IEEE Transactions on Artificial Intelligence, 2023.

[44] Karthick, G., Pankajavalli, P. and Pankajavalli, P. A review on human healthcare internet of things: A technical perspective. SN Computer Science, 1(4): 198, 2020.

[45] Hilty, D.M., Armstrong, C.M., Edwards-Stewart, A., Gentry, M.T., Luxton, D.D. and Krupinski, E.A. Sensor, wearable, and remote patient monitoring competencies for clinical care and training: Scoping review. Journal of Technology in Behavioral Science, 6: 252-277, 2021.

[46] Zeadally, S., Siddiqui, F., Baig, Z. and Ibrahim, A. Smart healthcare: Challenges and potential solutions using Internet of Things (IoT) and big data analytics. PSU Research Review, 4(2): 149-168, 2020.

[47] Akbarzadeh, O., Baradaran, M. and Khosravi, M.R. IoT-based smart management of healthcare services in hospital buildings during COVID-19 and future pandemics. Wireless Communications and Mobile Computing, 2021: 1-14, 2021.

[48] Dion, H., Evans, M. and Farrell, P. Hospitals management transformative initiatives: Towards energy efficiency and environmental sustainability in healthcare facilities. Journal of Engineering, Design and Technology, 21(2): 552-584, 2023.

[49] Shariaty, F., Caiqin, H., Pavlov, V.A., Duan, L., Zavyalov, S.V., Pervunina, T.M. and Ying, W. Integrating quantitative and convolutional features to enhance the efficiency of pathology classification in CT imaging. Computer Science, Telecommunications and Management, 16(4): 60-69, 2023.

[50] Mason, M., Cho, Y., Rayo, J., Gong, Y., Harris, M. and Jiang, Y. Technologies for medication adherence monitoring and technology assessment criteria: Narrative review. JMIR mHealth and uHealth, 10(3): e35157, 2022.

[51] Alftberg, Å. Medication management in Swedish nursing homes: An ethnographic study of resistance, negotiation and control. European Journal of Social Work, 25(2): 186-197, 2022.

[52] Šakić Trogrlić, R., van den Homberg, M., Budimir, M., McQuistan, C., Sneddon, A. and Golding, B. Early warning systems and their role in disaster risk reduction. Towards the "Perfect" Weather Warning: Bridging Disciplinary Gaps through Partnership and Communication, pp. 11-46. 2022. Springer International Publishing Cham.

[53] Marchezini, V., Horita, F.E.A., Matsuo, P.M., Trajber, R., Trejo-Rangel, M.A. and

Olivato, D. A review of studies on Participatory Early Warning Systems (P-EWS): Pathways to support citizen science initiatives. Frontiers in Earth Science, 6: 184, 2018.

[54] Kelman, I. and Glantz, M.H. Early warning systems defined. Reducing Disaster: Early Warning Systems for Climate Change, pp. 89-108, 2014.

[55] Roy, S.S., Roy, A., Samui, P., Gandomi, M. and Gandomi, A.H. Hateful sentiment detection in real-time tweets: An LSTM-based comparative approach. IEEE Transactions on Computational Social Systems, 2023.

[56] Ran, Y., Zhou, X., Lin, P., Wen, Y. and Deng, R. A survey of predictive maintenance: Systems, purposes and approaches. arXiv preprint arXiv:1912.07383, 2019.

[57] Feldmann, S., Buechele, R. and Preveden, V. Predictive maintenance – From data collection to value creation. Roland Berger GmbH, pp. 3-4, July, 2018.

[58] Matzka, S. Explainable artificial intelligence for predictive maintenance applications. *In:* 2020 Third International Conference on Artificial Intelligence for Industries (ai4i). 2020. IEEE.

[59] Scott, M.J., Verhagen, W.J., Bieber, M.T. and Marzocca, P.A. A systematic literature review of predictive maintenance for defence fixed-wing aircraft sustainment and operations. Sensors, 22(18): 7070, 2022.

[60] Kwame, A. and Petrucka, P.M. A literature-based study of patient-centered care and communication in nurse-patient interactions: Barriers, facilitators, and the way forward. BMC Nursing, 20(1): 1-10, 2021.

[61] Berntsen, G.R., Yaron, S., Chetty, M., Canfield, C., Ako-Egbe, L., Phan, P. et al. Person-centered care (PCC): The people's perspective. International Journal for Quality in Health Care, 33(Supplement_2): ii23-ii26, 2021.

[62] Butler, J.M., Gibson, B., Patterson, O.V., Damschroder, L.J., Halls, C.H., Denhalter, D.W. et al. Clinician documentation of patient centered care in the electronic health record. BMC Medical Informatics and Decision Making, 22(1): 1-12, 2022.

[63] Gartner, J.-B., Abasse, K.S., Bergeron, F., Landa, P., Lemaire, C. and Côté, A. Definition and conceptualization of the patient-centered care pathway, a proposed integrative framework for consensus: A concept analysis and systematic review. BMC Health Services Research, 22(1): 1-24, 2022.

[64] Edemekong, P.F., Annamaraju, P. and Haydel, M.J. Health Insurance Portability and Accountability Act. 2018.

[65] Bertino, E. Data security and privacy: Concepts, approaches, and research directions. *In:* 2016 IEEE 40th Annual Computer Software and Applications Conference (cOMPSAc). 2016. IEEE.

[66] Bandari, V. Enterprise data security measures: A comparative review of effectiveness and risks across different industries and organization types. International Journal of Business Intelligence and Big Data Analytics, 6(1): 1-11, 2023.

[67] Gupta, R., Saxena, D. and Singh, A.K. Data security and privacy in cloud computing: Concepts and emerging trends. arXiv preprint arXiv:2108.09508, 2021.

[68] Group, U.N.D. Data privacy, ethics and protection. Guidance Note on Big Data for Achievement of the 2030 Agenda. 2017.

[69] Koonrungsesomboon, N. and Hirayama, K. Ethical and regulatory challenges in genetic and genomic research involving stored biological specimens. Frontiers in Genetics, 13: 1062188, 2022.

[70] Sisk, B.A., Baldwin, K., Parsons, M. and DuBois, J.M. Ethical, regulatory, and practical barriers to COVID-19 research: A stakeholder-informed inventory of concerns. PloS One, 17(3): e0265252, 2022.

[71] Shariaty, F., Davydov, V., Yushkova, V., Glinushkin, A. and Rud, V.Y. Automated pulmonary nodule detection system in computed tomography images based on Active-contour and SVM classification algorithm. Journal of Physics: Conference Series. 2019. IOP Publishing.

[72] Roy, S.S., Krishna, P.V. and Yenduri, S. Analyzing intrusion detection system: An ensemble based stacking approach. *In:* 2014 IEEE International Symposium on Signal Processing and Information Technology (ISSPIT). 2014. IEEE.

[73] Wang, J., Liu, Y., Li, P., Lin, Z., Sindakis, S. and Aggarwal, S. Overview of data quality: Examining the dimensions, antecedents, and impacts of data quality. Journal of the Knowledge Economy, 1-20, 2023.

[74] Ehrlinger, L. and Wöß, W. A survey of data quality measurement and monitoring tools. Frontiers in Big Data, 5: 850611, 2022.

[75] Bandhu, A. and Roy, S.S. Classifying multi-category images using deep learning: A convolutional neural network model. *In:* 2017 2nd IEEE International Conference on Recent Trends in Electronics, Information & Communication Technology (RTEICT). 2017. IEEE.

[76] Newton, J.J., Data Element Naming Standards. 1998.

[77] Polito, C.C., Sevransky, J.E. and Dickert, N.W. Ethical and regulatory challenges in advancing prehospital research: Focus on sepsis. The American Journal of Emergency Medicine, 34(3): 623, 2016.

[78] Arora, K.S. and Blake, V. Uterus transplantation: Ethical and regulatory challenges. Journal of Medical Ethics, 40(6): 396-400, 2014.

[79] Curtis, R.G., Bartel, B., Ferguson, T., Blake, H.T., Northcott, C., Virgara, R. et al. Improving user experience of virtual health assistants: Scoping review. Journal of Medical Internet Research, 23(12): e31737, 2021.

[80] Agarwal, S., Agarwal, B. and Gupta, R. Chatbots and virtual assistants: A bibliometric analysis. Library Hi Tech, 40(4): 1013-1030, 2022.

[81] Alam, L. and Mueller, S. Examining the effect of explanation on satisfaction and trust in AI diagnostic systems. BMC Medical Informatics and Decision Making, 21(1): 178, 2021.

[82] Musalamadugu, T.S., Kumari, N. and Rodriquez, R.V. Impact of the AI-induced app 'Babylon' in the healthcare industry. *In:* Artificial Intelligence and Knowledge Processing, pp. 59-66. CRC Press.

[83] Prochaska, J.J., Vogel, E.A., Chieng, A., Kendra, M., Baiocchi, M., Pajarito, S. et al. A therapeutic relational agent for reducing problematic substance use (Woebot): Development and usability study. Journal of Medical Internet Research, 23(3): e24850, 2021.

[84] Chung, K. and Park, R.C. Chatbot-based heathcare service with a knowledge base for cloud computing. Cluster Computing, 22: 1925-1937, 2019.

[85] Steenkamer, B., de Weger, E., Drewes, H., Putters, K., Van Oers, H. and Baan, C. Implementing population health management: An international comparative study. Journal of Health Organization and Management, 34(3): 273-294, 2020.

[86] McShane, M. and Kirkham, K. Making it personal – Population health management and the NHS. Journal of Integrated Care, 28(3): 243-252, 2020.

[87] Alton, D.M. Population health management: From principal to practice. Journal of Integrated Care, 31(4), 2023.

[88] McCartney, G., Douglas, M., Taulbut, M., Katikireddi, S.V. and McKee, M. Tackling population health challenges as we build back from the pandemic. BMJ, 375, 2021.

[89] Roy, S.S., Hsu, C, Samaran, A., Goyal, R., Pande, A., Balas, V.E. et al. Vessels segmentation in angiograms using convolutional neural network: A deep learning based approach. CMES-Computer Modeling in Engineering & Sciences, 136(1): 241-255, 2023.

[90] Shariaty, F., Orooji, M., Mousavi, M., Baranov, M. and Velichko, E. Automatic lung segmentation in computed tomography images using active shape model. *In:* 2020 IEEE International Conference on Electrical Engineering and Photonics (EExPolytech). 2020. IEEE.

[91] Mousavi, M., Shariaty, F., Orooji, M. and Velichko, E. The performance of active-contour and region growing methods against noises in the segmentation of computed-tomography scans. *In:* International Youth Conference on Electronics, Telecommunications and Information Technologies: Proceedings of the YETI 2020, St. Petersburg, Russia. 2021. Springer.

[92] Schlender, J.F., Golden, A.G., Samant, T.S., Lagishetty, C.V. and Schmidt, S. The personalization of drug therapy for elderly patients. Developing Drug Products in an Aging Society: From Concept to Prescribing, 589-611, 2016.

[93] Iyer, P.M., Karthikeyan, S., Sanjay Kumar, P. and Krishnan Namboori, P. Comprehensive strategy for the design of precision drugs and identification of genetic signature behind proneness of the disease – A pharmacogenomic approach. Functional & Integrative Genomics, 17: 375-385, 2017.

[94] Laface, C. and Memeo, R. Clinical updates for gastrointestinal malignancies. MDPI, 1424, 2023.

[95] Roy, S.S. and Taguchi, Y. Handbook of Machine Learning Applications for Genomics. 2022. Springer.

[96] Levchuk, L.A., Roschina, O.V., Mikhalitskaya, E.V., Epimakhova, E.V., Simutkin, G.G., Bokhan, N.A. et al. Serum levels of S100B protein and myelin basic protein as a potential biomarkers of recurrent depressive disorders. Journal of Personalized Medicine, 13(9): 1423, 2023.

CHAPTER

6

IoT-powered AI for Precise Pneumonia Detection in Chest X-Rays

Sanjiban Sekhar Roy*, **Mohd Anas, Abhishek Kumar Pandey, Ramanathan L. and Kathiravan Srinivasan**

School of Computer Science and Engineering, Vellore Institute of Technology, Vellore 632014, India

In the ongoing battle against the global COVID-19 pandemic, IoT technology has been utilized to develop a revolutionary solution. A ground-breaking research study introduces an innovative technique for automatically and accurately classifying COVID-19 and normal pneumonia patients using chest X-ray images and IoT-based data. This innovation is centered around a specialized dilated convolutional neural network model meticulously designed to surpass the urgent need for precise diagnostics in similar lung conditions. The robustness and effectiveness of this approach have been extensively validated through comprehensive testing, highlighting its potential to transform COVID-19 diagnosis. The results proudly demonstrate an impressive 93% accuracy rate when evaluated with a standard chest X-ray dataset. Furthermore, as our data repository continues to expand, we anticipate even more remarkable advancements. In a world where COVID-19 data is limited compared to other prevalent diseases, our IoT-powered solution emerges as a beacon of hope, offering improved diagnostics and a pathway to more effective pandemic management. Amidst these challenging times, our research serves as evidence of the power of innovative technology and collective determination in the fight against the pandemic.

1. Introduction

The coronavirus disease 2019, commonly known as COVID-19, has become a global health crisis due to its highly infectious nature. "This is caused by

*Corresponding author: sanjibanroy09@gmail.com

the highly infectious and severe acute respiratory syndrome Coronavirus 2 (SARS-CoV-2)" [1]. Symptoms of this disease include difficulty in breathing, fever, and dry cough. Other associated symptoms include muscle pain, loss of smell, abdominal pain, and sore throat. While the majority of cases exhibit mild symptoms, a percentage of individuals may experience viral pneumonia and multi-organ failure as the disease progresses. As of April 30th, 2020, the COVID-19 pandemic has affected approximately 1.4 million people, with a global infection count of around 3.2 million [2]. Conventional techniques for diagnosing pneumonia are prone to subjectivity and heterogeneity among medical practitioners. In contrast, a standardized method for diagnosing pneumonia is offered by IoT-powered AI algorithms. These algorithms lessen subjectivity, which helps to guarantee consistent and trustworthy findings in a variety of contexts and reduce the possibility of misdiagnosis. IoT-powered AI systems offer several advantages over traditional methods for detecting coronavirus pneumonia in chest X-ray images. Chest X-rays can be analyzed in real-time with the help of these tools, which speeds up the process of diagnosis and treatment. Furthermore, these systems exhibit greater precision, especially during the initial phases of the illness. Lastly, they are less subjective, reducing the risk of misdiagnosis. The Internet of Things (IoT) has brought in the way physical objects interact with each other and share data over the Internet. This network of smart devices is embedded with sensors, software, and other cutting-edge technologies that allow seamless communication and data exchange between various systems and devices, making our lives more convenient and efficient. In the field of healthcare, IoT devices have gained prominence and have the potential to transform disease diagnosis and treatment, for diseases like COVID-19 included. Early detection of COVID-19 pneumonia via chest X-ray analysis is a potential use of IoT in healthcare. COVID-19 pneumonia is a severe complication of the COVID-19 virus that can be life-threatening if not promptly diagnosed and treated. Detecting COVID-19 early is crucial for optimal care. IoT-based systems are crucial in detecting COVID-19 pneumonia through automated analysis of chest X-ray images. In [38], the authors discuss the COVID-19 challenge and the need for precautionary measures without a vaccine. IoT devices generate extensive data, enabling data mining for virus detection. The authors' study employs a SVM and Artificial Bee Colony (ABC), achieving 95% prediction accuracy and demonstrating the value of dimensionality reduction in IoT data classification. With reference to [39], the COVID-19 pandemic highlights the critical need for fast and automated infection screening methods. Traditional methods like RT-PCR are costly and time-consuming, necessitating emerging AI and technology solutions. Combining 5G and IoT advancements in healthcare, this study introduces IoT-enabled neural network algorithms for coronavirus analysis with CT scans. Patient data is collected through IoT-enabled components and transmitted to a cloud server. IoT-powered AI can identify COVID pneumonia in X-rays by utilizing AI algorithms and sensors. Sensors collect data on X-ray properties like brightness, contrast, and texture, essential for the project. This data is then inputted into the AI algorithm, powered by deep learning algorithms. The AI algorithm analyzes the sensor data to identify patterns associated with COVID-19 pneumonia.

The following steps can achieve the overall objective of this work:

1. A patient's chest X-ray is taken by a digital X-ray machine.
2. The chest X-ray image is transmitted to an IoT-powered AI system using a wireless network.
3. The AI system analyzes the X-ray image and identifies any patterns associated with COVID-19 pneumonia.
4. If the AI system detects COVID-19 pneumonia, it alerts a radiologist.
5. The radiologist can then examine and confirm the diagnosis of the X-ray image.

The model, which consists of fine-tuned convolutional neural network stacked sub-models with a meta-learner, is evaluated on a dataset, demonstrating its effectiveness in detecting COVID-19 infections through CT scans.

1.1 Integration with IoT

This study aims to develop a CNN that can accurately distinguish between normal and COVID-19 pneumonia. It is important to note that integrating Internet of Things (IoT) concepts can enhance the capabilities and accuracy of diagnostic systems. IoT is the interconnection of hardware devices, communication technologies, and sensors that collect and exchange data over the Internet. In the context of healthcare and disease detection, facilitating real-time data acquisition and analysis, IoT can play a crucial role. Here, we introduce the concept of IoT in the context of our research objectives. The recent pandemic has had a catastrophic impact worldwide, causing millions of deaths. The need for automated and accurate diagnosis of COVID-19-affected patients globally. To enable automatic detection requires X-rays of chest images from infected patients exhibiting symptoms of common bacterial pneumonia, confirmed cases, and normal pneumonia patients. This study aims to develop an accurate method to classify COVID-19 and pneumonia chest X-ray images using IoT devices.

1.2 IoT-powered Diagnosis

In this era of interconnected devices, IoT can significantly enhance the diagnosis process by continuously monitoring patients' vital signs and symptoms. Smart wearable devices, such as IoT-enabled thermometers (such as MLX90614), pulse oximeter sensors (such as MAX30100), and respiratory rate monitors (such as ADXL345), can collect real-time health data from suspected COVID-19 patients. This data can be seamlessly integrated with the CNN-based diagnostic system, providing a holistic approach to patient assessment. Moreover, IoT devices can aid in remote patient monitoring, enabling healthcare professionals to track patients' progress and make timely interventions.

COVID-19 diagnosis relies on symptoms, history, and imaging tests like CT and X-ray scans [3]. Additionally, positive pathogenic testing is another way to identify COVID-19 patients. There have been cases where asymptomatic patients were detected as having normal pneumonia through CT scans, while pathogenic tests confirmed them as COVID-19 positive. Lower respiratory specimens, bronchoalveolar lavage, and sputum are usually collected for pathogenic testing [3, 4]. Computer-assisted image analysis has been a proven technique for better understanding images in recent years. Machine learning, especially deep learning, has made significant advancements in disease classification. Image segmentation can be done with higher accuracy using deep learning, which allows for more efficient feature extraction and learning [5, 47, 48].

Radiology has played a path-breaking role in diagnosing COVID-19 infections worldwide. Chest radiography helps identify asymmetric airspace opacities that contribute to the cause of coronavirus pneumonia [3]. The initial tests of COVID-19 patients often show bilateral lung involvement in 40 out of 41 cases. Various classification techniques based on convolutional neural networks (CNNs) have gained attention, as these deep learning-based methods offer better performance [6–11]. However, only a few classification methods related to CNNs have been proposed specifically for coronavirus images [12–15]. Previous versions of CNN techniques in the literature have overlooked the activation of parameters and the criticality of local features. Randomly increasing the dilation rate should also be avoided, as it may affect feature collection. Our proposed method, named dilated convolutional neural network, achieves an accuracy of 87% in classifying normal and COVID-19 pneumonia.

Though some methods based on convolutional neural networks achieve high levels of accuracy, the layers involved in data processing can be time-consuming. Additionally, the small receptive field in CNNs often leads to poor accuracy. Therefore, effective feature extraction requires a different technique. Another drawback is that recent versions of CNN models have not focused on parameter activation . To address these issues, the proposed dilated convolutional model with increasing dilation rates reduces sparsity in the dilated feature map, allowing for more context extraction from the analyzed image area. A simple CNN typically consists of convolutional layers, with each layer resulting in a linear increase in the receptive field. However, this linear growth limits the performance of traditional CNNs on input images [16]. Due to the recent pandemic, limited research has been conducted on using machine learning or deep learning to classify X-rays. To enhance the accuracy of our diagnostic model, we propose integrating IoT-based data into the training and validation process. Real-time data collected from IoT devices can capture dynamic changes in patients' health conditions, resulting in a more robust and adaptable CNN model, which is crucial in a rapidly evolving pandemic scenario.

Our developed method has achieved favorable results compared to other existing methods in the literature, utilizing an available COVID-19 dataset. However, due to the sensitive nature of the issue and the current conditions, there is a scarcity of COVID-19 data compared to other common lung conditions. In Figure 2, we illustrate a potential integration of IoT devices for COVID-19 detection. In the future, once the research community can collect and curate a sufficiently large dataset on COVID-19, the proposed model will be further evaluated. The aim of this study is to develop a deep learning model that can accurately detect COVID-19 pneumonia patients from a dataset of chest X-ray images supported by the Internet of Things. Our method utilizes a dilated deep convolutional neural network approach. The research outcome can be integrated into larger diagnostic systems to assist physicians and radiologists in achieving better and earlier diagnoses.

The rest of this article is structured in the following manner: Section 2 discusses recent developments in CNN-based applications for COVID-19 X-ray images. In Section 3, we introduce our proposed methodology. Section 4 details the dataset, data augmentation method, activation maps of hidden layers, and comparative analysis of experimental outcomes. The article is concluded in Section 5 and future work is outlined.

2. Related Work

Deep learning methods have found prominence and have been the pioneers in image classification and segmentation tasks. Various types of image-related problems, such as brain MRI images [17], chest X-rays, and retina-related problems, have found their solutions using deep learning, especially CNN [18, 19]. X-ray images are cheap and used to scan numerous organs faster in the hospital. Singh and colleagues, in their 2020 study, explored the advantages of IoT in swiftly recognizing symptoms and improving treatment for individuals affected by COVID-19. This technology proves beneficial not only to patients but also extends its advantages to medical practitioners, surgeons, and the efficient management of healthcare facilities [43]. The study in [41] uses big data analysis with TEXTOM to compare pre-pandemic (Jan 2018-2019) and pandemic (Jan 2020-Dec 2021) periods, revealing trends in the fitness and healthcare industries, including common themes like fitness, research, smart management, and future technology, as well as distinct clusters. The proposed model's prime idea is to train the COVID-19 pneumonia X ray images using deep learning, especially CNN, which would be a great help to medical experts in diagnosing COVID-19 patients. The authors in [14] have proposed Inception- ResNetV2 and InceptionV3 for classifications of chest X-ray radiographs [20]. They have provided ROC analyses and confusion matrices; however, their confusion matrices have provided false negative and false positive values as zero, which signifies a perfect test. However, this is not possible and may signify a data imbalance problem. In [40], the authors have stated that the rise of IoT applications in recent years has provided innovative solutions to various challenges, and their paper introduces a machine learning-enabled smart IoT-based application for diagnosing brain hemorrhages, achieving an accuracy of 80.67% with SVM and 86.7% with artificial neural networks, offering valuable diagnostic support and educational benefits for radiologists. In Atawi et al. [42] it is shown how IoT's sensor-based devices can offer a brilliant technique to lower the risk of surgery in the complex situation of health care, especially during COVID-19.

A transfer learning model has been proposed very recently by [15] that claimed to have detected various abnormalities in tiny X-ray images [13]. They have obtained accuracy, sensitivity, and specificity. A handfulof work on the COVID-19 crisis also has been accessed from a pathological point of view, such as in Xu et al. [21]. Wong et al. have found the frequency and distribution of chest radiographs [14, 46]. Visual Geometry Group Network (VGG19) and Google Mobile Net have been incorporated into the work of Hemadan et al. [15]. However, this work still needs to provide activation maps, which we have obtained in our proposed method.

Barstugan et al. [22] have classified CT images by support vector machines (SVM). They have used maximal 10-fold cross-validations [23]. In this work, the authors have considered common bacterial pneumonia, confirmed COVID-19 cases, and normal pneumonia so that classification can be carried out using transfer learning. Using transfer learning, different abnormalities in a small image could also be achieved; that is what the authors believed and successfully achieved good results also. The authors also have referred to the literature, where VGG19, MobileNet v2, Inception, Inception ResNet v2, and Xception models were used and have compared their results with these models. Authors have decided on the parameter after many experiments and have referred that a handful of contributions could be possible in the future. They have found sensitivity, specificity, precision, accuracy, and F_1 score values. Barstugan et al. [24] have proposed a capsule network for classifying X-ray Images. Other works can also be identified in the recent literature [25–27].

3. The Proposed Method

Image classification is a common application of convolutional neural networks, contributing immensely to medical diagnosis in recent times. Assuming G is discrete [16], $G : Z^2 \leftarrow R$. Lets further assume $Q_r = [-r, r]^2 \cap Z^2$ and $k = Q_r \leftarrow R$ is $(2r+1)^2$ filter size. The convolution operator $*$ can be written as $(F * k)(p) = \Sigma_{s+t=p} F(s)k(t)$. Further, we can propose a generalizing l and dilation rate l we can further define $(F_l k)(p) = \Sigma_{s+p} F(s)k(t)$. When the dilation rate l=1, the network is a simple convolutional neural network. In the literature, the theorem of convolution, which is primarily related to the Fourier transform, has been mentioned by a handful of authors in the past. Moreover, this also can be referred to as Fast Fourier Transformation (FFT) [28–33].

$$f(x) = h \oplus g = \int_{-\alpha}^{\alpha} h(x-u)g(u)du = F^{-1}(\sqrt{2\pi}F[h]F[g]) \tag{1}$$

The symbol ⊕ refers to the convolution operation. F and F^{-1} refer to the Fourier transform and inverse Fourier transform F^{-1}, respectively. $\sqrt{2\pi}$ signifies a constant. Equation (3) presents the convolution theorem, g, and h is a convolution of two continuous functions, and the final hypothesis is $f(x)$. Here, g signifies the kernel function, and h is the input image. The activation map, also referred to as the feature map, output of a filter applied to the previous layer in a convolutional neural network. The mathematical equation of feature map is given below:

$$FM = \text{input} \oplus \text{kernel} = \sum_{k=0}^{col} \sum_{x=0}^{row} \text{input}(x-a, k-b) = F^{-1}\,(\sqrt{2\pi}F[h]F[g]) \tag{2}$$

$\oplus FF^{-1}\sqrt{2\pi}$ at (i, j) in the mth feature matrix of lth layer i.e. $z^{l}_{i,j,m}$ can be represented in equation 3.

$$z^{l}_{i,j,m} = w^{l^T}_{m} + b^{l}_{m} \tag{3}$$

The representation of weight vector w^{l}_{m} and bias is b^{l}_{m}. The input can be represented as x^{l}_{i} at location (i, j). Activation function is $a(\cdot)$; in the case of a CNN, it is represented as $a^{l}_{i,j.m}$. It can be given as, $a^{l}_{i,j.m}$. The function can be referred as *pooling* $(\cdot)$ and for every feature map, we can refer the pooling function as, $y^{l}_{i,j.m}$ = *pooling* $(a^{l}_{p,q.m})$, for all (p, q) ε $R_{i,j}$.

Algorithm 1 Dilated deep convolutional neural network.

Input: COVID-19 Image dataset
Output: Trained COVID-19 classifier
Initialization CNN using random weights
  Accuracy ← 0
  for *epoch steps* = 1, 2,3, ..., N_{epochs} **do**
    for *X-rayimage* = 1, 2,3 ..., $N_{batchsize}$ **do**
      X-ray *Image*$_{data}$ ← *Resizing*(X-ray *Image*)
        Image$_{data}$ ← *Augmentation(Image)*
        Inputlayer ← *Image*$_{data}$
        // neural network hidden layers
      High *dilation_factor* features
      Low *dilation factor* fine map
      $w(t)$ output layer return diagnosed results
      Calculate *Binary cross entropy loss*
      Update back propagation weights for Use
      Adam Optimized to min $e(t)$
    end
  end
Evaluate the model using various classification metrics.

3.1 Dilated CNN Classification Model

In the case of the dilated CNN, an additional parameter known as the dilation rate is introduced [34, 35]. In this study, the conventional CNN is configured to extract more information from X-ray images of COVID-19 at each convolutional layer. Using the smallest 3×3 filters in all directions (up, down, right, left), a 3×3 convolutional layer is employed to extract detailed features from COVID-19 X-ray images. By using dilation in the CNN layers, the model is able to extract such features without the need for larger filters of size 5×5, which would result in additional computational overhead, and are typically used for detecting coarse-level features like shapes and contours.

Figure 1 represents the architecture of the dilated CNN. Our proposed architecture consists of 4 convolutional layers and 3 pooling layers, followed by dense and densely connected layers. This neural network is trained on RGB images with (128, 128, 3) shapes. The proposed dilated CNN layers utilize a fixed 3x3 filter, and the size of the receptive field is controlled by the dilation rate. Conv1 generates 32 feature maps in the first layer at a dilation of 2 with the ReLU activation function. The subsequent layer, Conv2, also uses a dilation rate of 2 with the ReLU activation function and generates 32 feature maps. The following convolutional layer, Conv3, employs a dilation rate of 2 with the ReLU function, producing 64 feature maps. In the last layer, Conv4 has a dilation rate of 2 and generates 32 feature maps.

The pooling layers combine the generated feature maps based on a user-defined rule, such as Max, Min, and Mean. In this model, 3 Max pooling layers

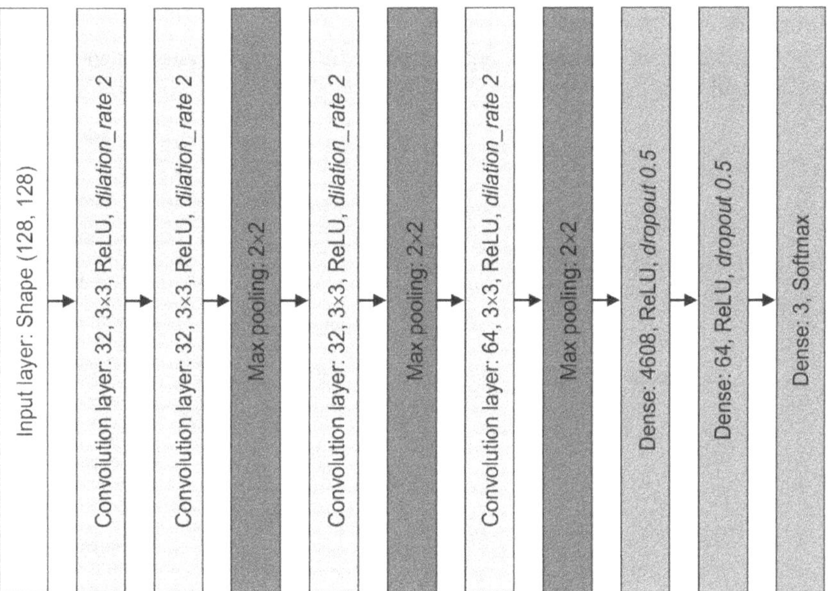

Figure 1. The architecture of the proposed dilated convolution neural network model

are placed after Conv1, Conv2, and Conv3. Both MaxPool1 and MaxPool2 are defined with a pool size of 2×2. After pooling, the features are flattened before being connected to the dense, fully connected layers. The Dense1 layer consists of 64 nodes with the ReLU activation function. The Dense2 layer consists of 64 units and utilizes the ReLU activation function. Both layers are followed by a dropout rate of 50% to prevent overfitting on the relatively small dataset. The output layer comprises 3 nodes using the softmax function, as it is a multi-class classification. The model is trained for 10 epochs with the Adam optimizer to minimize categorical cross-entropy loss (Algorithm 1).

3.2 IoT-enabled Data Integration

To further enhance the accuracy of our diagnostic model, we propose integrating IoT-based data into the training and validation process. Real-time data collected from IoT devices can be incorporated into the model to capture dynamic changes in a patient's health conditions. Vital signs and other health indicators can be tracked by wearable IoT devices, such as fitness trackers and smartwatches. Metrics, including body temperature, oxygen saturation levels, breathing rate, and heart rate, can be monitored by these gadgets. These wearables' real-time data can offer insightful information about a person's health, including any possible COVID-19 symptoms. IoT devices' real-time data can be integrated with the COVID X-ray image dataset in the Google Cloud Data Fusion. This integration can lead to a more robust and adaptable CNN model, which is crucial in a rapidly evolving pandemic scenario. In Figure 2 below, we present a probable architecture of neural network-based models and an IoT-based healthcare system to identify COVID-19 patients.

To enhance the accuracy of our diagnostic model, we proposed incorporating IoT-derived data in the training and validation process. This integration opens

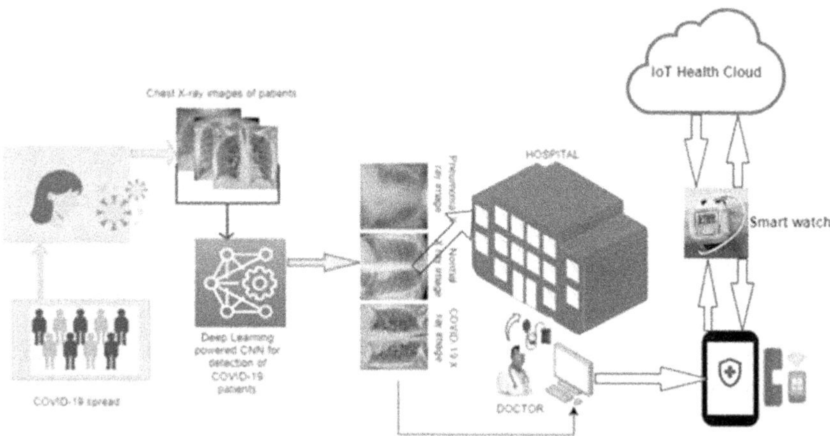

Figure 2. IoT-powered AI detects COVID-19 pneumonia in chest X-rays

new dimensions of real-time patient monitoring and healthcare intelligence. By incorporating real-time data collected from a network of IoT devices, our model becomes proficient in capturing dynamic changes in patients' health conditions. This capability offers timely and context-aware insights that are crucial for managing a rapidly evolving pandemic scenario. The inclusion of IoT-driven insights enhances the adaptability and robustness of our CNN model, ensuring it remains at the forefront of precision diagnostics. Figure 2 illustrates our envisioned objectives. This demonstrates the promising future of intelligent healthcare solutions. Subsequently, advanced analytics can be utilized to recognize trends, identify epidemics, and forecast the spread of diseases. Decision-makers and healthcare professionals can view this information in an easily navigable style using the data visualization tools on their smartphones or computers. It's important to note that this entire architecture represents a possible use case. In this scenario, the smartwatch continuously tracks the user's vital signs, including pulse, blood oxygen, blood pressure, and heart rate. The data is then streamed in real-time to a cloud-based health management platform.

4. Experimental Results

4.1 Description of Dataset

This image dataset is a collection of 1288 chest X-rays collected and curated as part of the open-source Kaggle image dataset "https://www.kaggle.com/datasets/prashant268/chest-xray-covid19-pneumonia". The aim of the experiment is to help identify general pneumonia and COVID-19 pneumonia, and to propose a model that learns the specific features that differentiate COVID-19 from pneumonia. The control set of 855 pneumonia images is sampled from the open-source chest X-ray image dataset, which is provided by the National Institutes of Health [36]. All images contain the Posteroanterior (PA) view of the patient's chest. The chest X-rays of patients with pneumonia are normal and are presented in Figures 3a, 3b, and 3c, respectively.

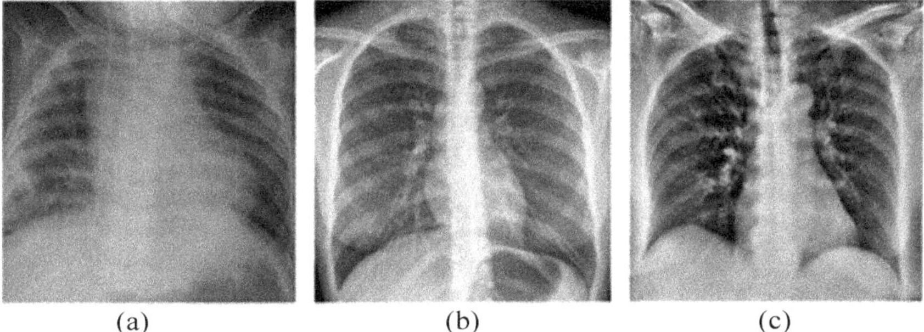

Figure 3. Chest X-ray of patients with (a) Pneumonia, (b) Normal, and (c) COVID-19

4.2 Data Augmentation

The functionality of deep learning algorithms is heavily reliant on data. The size of the network is proportional to the amount of data, such as images. When the available data is insufficient, the model can overfit and memorize the dataset. As a result, the model performs poorly on unseen test data as it fails to generalize well. To prevent overfitting and creating a reliable model for classifying X-ray images related to COVID-19, the images are augmented using the Keras image data generator with user-defined parameters. The augmentation techniques include a rotation of 10 degrees to change the orientation around the axis, random width shift and height shift of up to 10% of image dimensions, a shear range of 0.1 to distort the image shear, and a zoom of 0.1. The images can only be flipped horizontally around the y-axis to create symmetrical mirror images. Vertical flip is not possible for these images. Figure 4 illustrates the data augmentation process. All images are of the Posterior-Anterior (PA) view, where the patient is X-rayed while lying on their back. This view captures both the left and right lungs of the patient. Due to the lung structure, the images can only be flipped around the vertical axis [18, 19, 37, 44, 45]. The augmented data can be fed to IoT (Internet of Things) devices through various methods and technologies to enhance their functionality and decision-making capabilities. Here are several ways this can be achieved:

(a) Data Integration Platforms: Utilizing middleware or integration platforms such as Google Cloud Data Fusion to merge augmented data with IoT device data streams for compatibility.
(b) Cloud Services: Opting for cloud platforms to store, process, and deliver augmented data to IoT devices, thereby enhancing their functionality.
(c) APIs and Web Services: Developing APIs or web services to transmit augmented data in real-time to IoT devices, enabling seamless integration.
(d) Edge Computing: Implementing edge computing solutions to process and augment data closer to the IoT device, reducing latency.
(e) Sensor Enhancements and AI: Deploying advanced sensors on the IoT device to capture more data, while employing AI for analysis and decision-making based on augmented data.

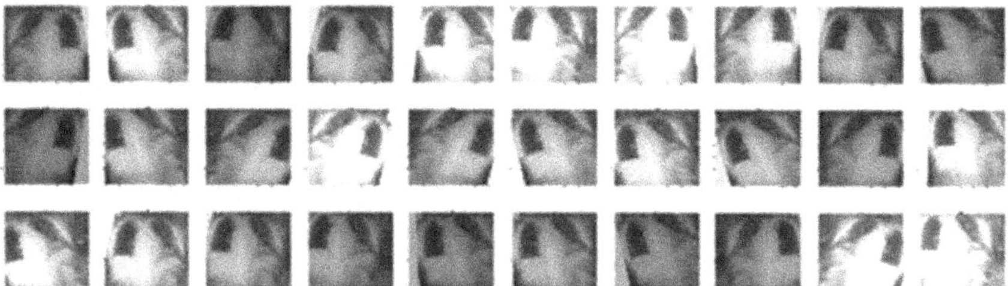

Figure 4. Data augmentation helps to introduce some degree of randomness for X-ray input images after applying horizontal flip, brightness, sheer, zoom, shift, and rotation

4.3 Activation Functions

In this proposed work, all the hidden layers have used an activation function called ReLU. It avoids saturation and offers more sensitivity towards the sums of activations. This function is nonlinear by nature. However, it looks like a linear function. Using non-linearity, it learns complex relations. It is a part of a wiser linear function that learns half of the input domain as linear, and another part of the input domain is learned as a non-linear function. The final outcome layer helps predict the output of multi-class classification. In this work, the softmax activation function has been chosen. The validity of the CNN can be checked using feature maps. In addition, feature maps signify the active areas of the images. In this study, the highlighted areas of the images have contributed to the COVID-19 patients' X-ray classifications, and they are shown in the feature maps below for all stages of the convolutional layers. In Figure 4, we represent each layer of the dilated CNN with activation maps.

The feature maps in Figure 5 (a, b, c, d) show results from different convolution and pooling layers. Based on the dilation rate, we can absorb that

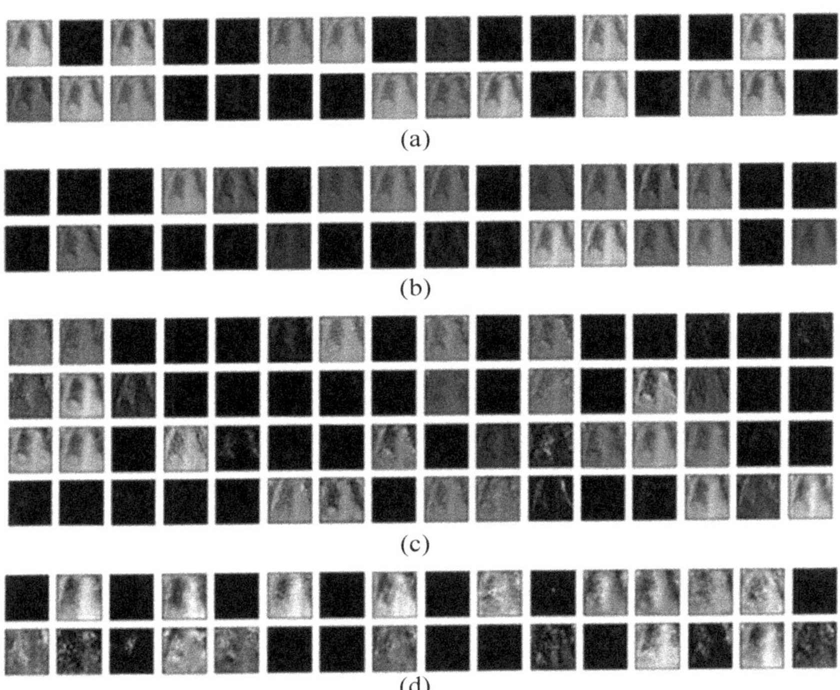

Figure 5. Activation maps for various layers of the Dilated CNN. Each of the three convolutional layers depicts the granularityof the generated features, with coarse features generated in Conv1 and fine features in Conv3. The MaxPooling layers reduce the resolution of the generated features using a 2×2 kernel

the convolution layers with higher dilation rates, i.e., 4 and 2 (Conv1 and Conv2), focus on the coarse features and the layer Conv3 with a dilation rate of 1 (equal to basic convolution) generates features of fine granularity in comparison. The flattened features are connected to fully connected dense layers. In the final last layer contains a one node and utilizes a softmax activation for multi-class classification. The following dilated CNN has been proposed for classifying X-ray images of patients.

The training accuracy plot is shown in Figure 6. The lack of data makes it difficult to build a model that will generalize well. To prevent such an issue and the model from over-fitting, many data augmentations are applied. These augmentations include rotation (5 degrees), width shift (10%), brightness range [0.5, 1.5], height shift (10%), shear range (0.1), and horizontal flip. Due to the images having only one axis of rotation (left to right and right to left rotation), a vertical flip is impossible. The training accuracy experiences small fluctuations due to dataset size and augmentation techniques. Figure 7

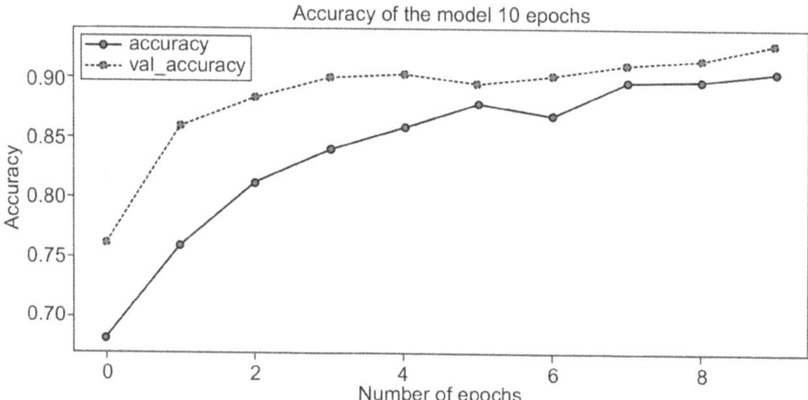

Figure 6. Model validation and training accuracy over 10 epochs

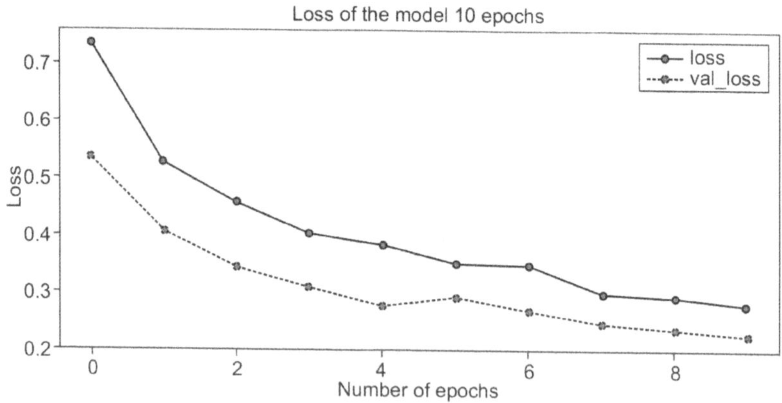

Figure 7. Model validation and training loss over 10 epochs

shows that while the validation loss plateaus, the training loss decreases. The Adam optimizer is utilized with the categorical cross-entropy loss function to train the model. The Y-axis denotes the binary cross entropy loss value, while X-axis represents the number of training epochs.

It can be observed from Table 1 that the dilated convolutional neural network achieved high accuracy.

Table 1. Classification performance of the proposed dilated CNN model

	Precision	Recall	F_1 score	Support
COVID-19	0.98	0.88	0.93	116
Normal	0.87	0.88	0.88	317
Pneumonia	0.94	0.96	0.95	855
Accuracy			0.93	1288
Micro avg	0.93	0.90	0.92	1288
Weighted avg	0.93	0.93	0.93	1288

Table 2. Classification performance of the traditional CNN model

	Precision	Recall	F_1 score	Support
COVID-19	0.95	0.82	0.88	116
Normal	0.87	0.89	0.81	317
Pneumonia	0.94	0.89	0.92	855
Accuracy			0.89	1288
Micro avg	0.88	0.87	0.87	1288
Weighted avg	0.89	0.89	0.89	1288

(CNN) is 93%. For the experiment, we divided the data into a training set and a holdout test set to ensure reliable results. one for training the model (80%) and another for testing (20%). According to Table 2, the accuracy of a traditional CNN is 89%, which is slightly lower than that of the proposed dilated CNN. Utilization of the Dilated CNN for classification provides a more comprehensive understanding of the results, particularly in the context of medical analysis. Metrics such as accuracy may not present the complete picture. Instead, metrics like recall, F1 score, and precision show how the approach performs on the holdout test set. When it comes to classifying COVID-19 patients from the data, the recall metric is crucial as it categorizes the relevant COVID-19 cases. The table demonstrates that the neural network model achieved a high precision (0.98) and high recall (0.88) for COVID-19 classification, both of which are desirable characteristics. For pneumonia classification, the precision and recall values were also high, with precision at 0.94 and recall at 0.96. Since both precision and recall values are comparable and similar, the F1 score is also high: COVID-19 (0.93) and Pneumonia (0.88). Additionally, the model is capable of detecting cases where there is no medical condition that is labeled as "normal." The recall (0.88), F1 score (0.88), and precision (0.87) for these cases are high. COVID-19 and pneumonia X-ray images can be accurately differentiated, enabling the correct classification of most data points. The confusion matrix for the proposed and traditional CNN are represented in Figures 8 and 9, respectively.

4.4 Comparative Performance

The following works have been published in which researchers have utilized neural network techniques to aid in identifying COVID-19 from CT scans and X-ray images. In ref. [2], 3D CT scans were employed, and a solution was presented to classify and screen COVID-19 cases. The dataset comprised CT scan images collected from patients, categorized as either COVID-19 negative or positive. In this binary classification problem, the paper states that they achieved a validation accuracy of 89.5% and an external validation accuracy of 85.25%, with a specificity of 0.88 and sensitivity of 0.87. Another research effort from the University of Waterloo introduced a model named "COVID-Net" [3]. The researchers conducted a multi-class classification task using chest X-ray images to distinguish between COVID-19, pneumonia, and normal cases. The authors achieved an accuracy of 92.6% with a COVID-19 sensitivity of 87.1% and a positive predicted value of 96.4% [13]. Due to limited COVID-19 data availability, only 31 images were used in the testing dataset.

4.5 Future Directions with IoT

As the IoT ecosystem continues to evolve and expand, incorporating advanced IoT technologies into COVID-19 diagnosis will remain a promising avenue for research. By leveraging real-time data from IoT devices, not only can diagnostic accuracy be enhanced, but valuable insights into disease progression and patient management can also be obtained. This, in turn, will contribute to more effective healthcare solutions in pandemic situations.

1. COVID-19 Detection utilizing Deep Learning: Limited research is available on using neural network techniques to classify COVID-19 from CT scans and X-rays. Notably, a few papers have explored the use of 3D CT scans for classifying COVID-19 patients. The dataset comprises CT scan images categorized as COVID-19 negative and positive.
2. Multi-Class Classification: The University of Waterloo has introduced COVID-Net, a model that can categorize COVID-19, pneumonia, and normal patient.

These research endeavors indicate promising directions for applying deep learning and multi-class classification techniques in IoT-based COVID-19 diagnosis. Acquiring a comprehensive and diverse dataset is crucial for ensuring the robustness and generalizability of machine learning models in real-world healthcare settings.

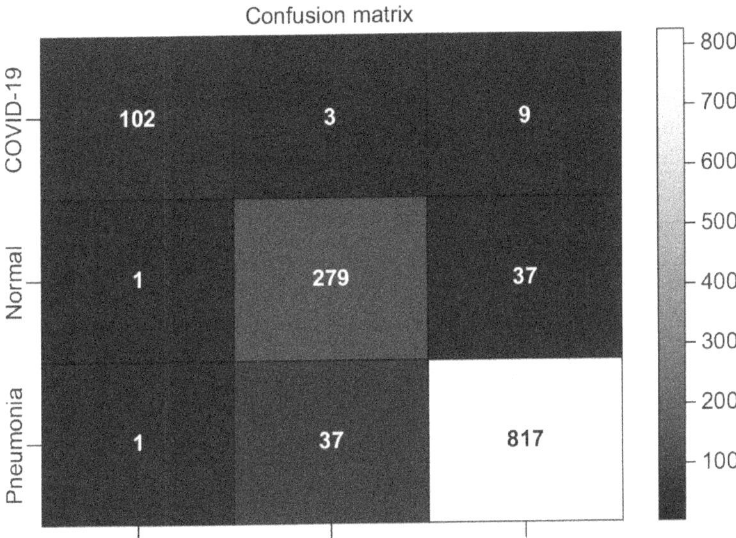

Figure 8. Confusion matrix of the proposed dilated CNN model

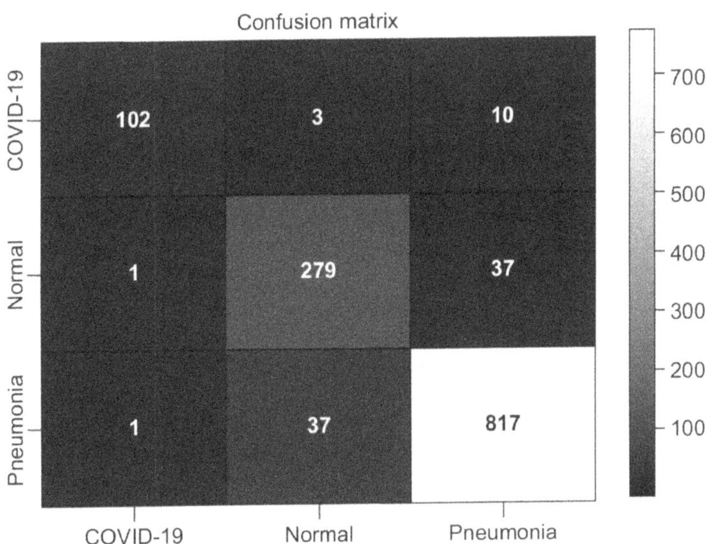

Figure 9. Confusion matrix of the traditional CNN model

5. Conclusions and Future Work

Amid the ongoing global struggle against the COVID-19 pandemic, we have harnessed the immense potential of Internet of Things (IoT) technology to develop a solution. Our innovative research introduces a novel method for the automatic and precise identification of COVID-19 pneumonia patients based on chest X-ray images and IoT-based data. At the heart of this innovation is a specialized dilated CNN model, meticulously crafted to meet and surpass the urgent need for accurate diagnostics, especially in the presence of similar lung conditions. The robustness and effectiveness of our approach have been rigorously confirmed through comprehensive testing, underscoring its potential to revolutionize the landscape of COVID-19 diagnosis. We take pride in the fact that our results exhibit an impressive 93% accuracy rate when assessed with a standard chest X-ray dataset. Moreover, as our data repository continues to expand, we anticipate even more significant improvements ahead. In a world where COVID-19 data is relatively scarce in comparison to other prevalent diseases, our IoT-powered solution emerges as a ray of hope, promising not only enhanced diagnostics but also a path to more effective pandemic management. As we navigate these challenging times, our research stands as a testament to the transformative power of cutting-edge technology and collective determination in the ongoing battle against the pandemic.

References

[1] Wang, H., Paulson, K.R., Pease, S.A., Watson, S.H., Comfort, P., Zheng, A.Y. et al. Estimating excess mortality due to the COVID-19 pandemic: A systematic analysis of COVID-19-related mortality, 2020–21. The Lancet, 399(10334): 1513-1536, 2022.

[2] Hosseiny, M., Kooraki, S., Gholamrezanezhad, A., Reddy, S., Myers, L. et al. Radiology perspective of coronavirus disease 2019 (Covid-19): Lessons from severe acute respiratory syndrome and middle east respiratory syndrome. American Journal of Roentgenology, 214(5): 1078-1082, 2020. doi:10.2214/ajr.20.22969.

[3] Chen, N., Zhou, M., Dong, X., Qu, J., Gong, F. Han, Y. et al. Epidemiological and clinical characteristics of 99 cases of 2019 novel coronavirus pneumonia in Wuhan, China: A descriptive study. The Lancet, 395(10223): 507-513, 2020. doi:10.1016/s0140-6736(20)30211-7.

[4] Bekhet, S., Alkinani, M.H., Tabares-Soto, R. and Hassaballah, M. An efficient method for (COVID-19) detection using light weight convolutional neural network. Computers, Materials and Continua, 69(2): 2021. 2475-2491.

[5] Arteaga-Arteaga, H.B., Mora-Rubio, A., Bravo-Ortíz, M.A., Alzate-Grisales, J.A., Arias-Garzón, D., López-Murillo, L.H. et al. Deep learning applied to Covid-19 detection in X-ray images. AI Applications for Disease Diagnosis and Treatment, IGI Global, pp. 202-247, 2022.

[6] Afshar, P., Mohammadi, A. and Plataniotis, K.N. Brain tumor type classification via capsule networks. 2018. doi:10.48550/ARXIV.1802.10200. https://arxiv.org/abs/1802.10200.

[7] Bekhet, S., Hassaballah, M., Kenk, M.A. and Hameed, M.A. An artificial intelligence based technique for COVID-19 diagnosis from chest X-ray. In: 2nd Novel Intelligent and Leading Emerging Sciences Conference (NILES), pp. 191-195, 2020. IEEE.

[8] L. S.K., S.N. Mohanty, S.K., A.N., Ramirez, G. Optimal deep learning model for classification of lung cancer on CT images. Future Generation Computer Systems, 92: 374-382, 2019. doi:https://doi.org/10.1016/j.future.2018.10.009. https://www.sciencedirect.com/science/article/pii/S0167739X18317011

[9] Hemanth, D.J., Anitha, J., Naaji, A., Geman, O., Popescu, D.E. and Hoang Son, L. A modified deep convolutional neural network for abnormal brain image classification. IEEE Access, 7: 4275-4283, 2019. doi:10.1109/ACCESS.2018.2885639.

[10] Afshar, P., Plataniotis, K.N. and Mohammadi, A. Capsule networks for brain tumor classification based on MRI images and coarse tumor boundaries. In: ICASSP 2019 – 2019 IEEE International Conference on Acoustics, Speech and Signal Processing (ICASSP), pp. 1368-1372, 2019. doi:10.1109/ICASSP.2019.8683759.

[11] Yu, F. and Koltun, V. Multi-scale context aggregation by dilated convolutions. 2015. doi:10.48550/ARXIV.1511.07122. https://arxiv.org/abs/1511.07122

[12] Lin, G., Wu, Q., Qiu, L. and Huang, X. Image super-resolution using a dilated convolutional neural network. Neurocomputing, 275: 1219-1230, 2018. doi:https://doi.org/10.1016/j.neucom.2017.09.062.https://www.sciencedirect.com/science/article/pii/S0925231217315813

[13] Wang, S., Kang, B., Ma, J., Zeng, X., Xiao, M., Guo, J. et al. A deep learning algorithm using CT images to screen for corona virus disease (Covid-19). European Radiology, 2021.doi:10.1007/s00330-021-07715-1.

[14] Narin, A., Kaya, C. and Pamuk, Z. Automatic detection of coronavirus disease (Covid-19) using X-ray imagesand deep convolutional neural networks. Pattern Analysis and Applications, 24(3): 1207-1220, 2021. doi:10.1007/s10044-021-00984-y.

[15] Apostolopoulos, I.D. and Mpesiana, T.A. Covid-19: Automatic detection from X-ray images utilizing transfer learning with convolutional neural networks. Physical and Engineering Sciences in Medicine, 43(2): 635-640, 2020. doi:10.1007/s13246-020-00865-4.

[16] Yu, F. and Koltun, V. Multi-scale context aggregation by dilated convolutions. 2015. doi:10.48550/ARXIV.1511.07122. https://arxiv.org/abs/1511.07122

[17] Abd-Ellah, M.K., Awad, A.I., Khalaf, A.A. and Hamed, H.F. A review on brain tumor diagnosis from MRI images: Practical implications, key achievements, and lessons learned. Magnetic Resonance Imaging, 61: 300-318, 2019. doi:https://doi.org/10.1016/j.mri.2019.05.028.

[18] Mahmud, M., Kaiser, M.S. and Hussain, A. Deep learning in mining biological data. 2020. doi:10.48550/ ARXIV.2003.00108. https://arxiv.org/abs/2003.00108

[19] Mahmud, M., Kaiser, M.S., Hussain, A. and Vassanelli, S. Applications of deep learning and reinforcement learning to biological data. IEEE Transactions on Neural Networks and Learning Systems, 29(6): 2063-2079, 2018. doi:10.1109/tnnls.2018.2790388.

[20] Wootton, D. and Feldman, C. The diagnosis of pneumonia requires a chest radiograph (X-ray) – Yes, no or sometimes. Pneumonia, 5(S1): 1-7, 2014. doi:10.15172/pneu.2014.5/464.

[21] Dai, Y. and Zhuang, P. Compressed sensing MRI via a multi-scale dilated residual convolution network. Magnetic Resonance Imaging, 63: 93-104, 2019. doi:https://doi.org/10.1016/j.mri.2019.07.014.https://www.sciencedirect.com/science/article/pii/S0730725X19301547

[22] Xu, Z., Shi, L., Wang, Y., Zhang, J., Huang, L., Zhang, C. et al. Pathological findings of Covid-19 associated with acute respiratory distress syndrome. The Lancet Respiratory Medicine, 8(4): 420-422, 2020. doi:10.1016/s2213-2600(20)30076-x.

[23] Wong, H.Y., Lam, H.Y., Fong, A.H.-T., Leung, S.T., Chin, T.W.-Y., Lo, C.S. et al. Frequency and distribution of chest radiographic findings in patients positive for Covid-19. Radiology, 296(2): 2020. doi:10.1148/radiol.2020201160.

[24] Hemdan, E.E.-D., Shouman, M.A. and Karar, M.E. Covidx-net: A framework of deep learning classifiers to diagnose Covid-19 in X-ray images. 2020. doi:10.48550/ARXIV.2003.11055. https://arxiv.org/abs/2003.11055

[25] Barstugan, M., Ozkaya, U. and Ozturk, S. Coronavirus (COVID-19) classification using CT images by machine learning methods. 2020. doi:10.48550/ARXIV.2003.09424. https://arxiv.org/abs/2003.09424

[26] Pham, Q.-V., Nguyen, D.C., Huynh-The, T., Hwang, W.-J. and Pathirana, P.N. Artificial intelligence (AI) and big data for coronavirus (Covid-19) pandemic: A survey on the state-of-the-arts. IEEE Access, 8: 130820-130839, 2020.. doi:10.1109/ACCESS.2020.3009328.

[27] Xu, X., Jiang, X., Ma, C., Du, P., Li, X., Lv, S. et al. A deep learning system to screennovel coronavirus disease 2019 pneumonia. Engineering, 6(10): 1122-1129, 2020. doi:10.1016/j.eng. 2020.04.010. https://doi.org/10.10162Fj.eng.2020.04.010

[28] Gudigar, A., Raghavendra, U., Nayak, S., Ooi, C.P., Chan, W.Y., Gangavarapu, M.R. et al. Role of artificial intelligence in Covid-19 detection. Sensors,21(23): 8045, 2021. doi:10.3390/s21238045.

[29] Alimadadi, A., Aryal, S., Manandhar, I., Munroe, P.B., Joe, B., Cheng, X. et al. Artificial intelligence and machine learning to fight Covid-19. Physiological Genomics, 52(4): 200-202, 2020. doi:10.1152/ physiolgenomics.00029.2020.

[30] Lin, G., Wu, Q., Qiu, L. and Huang, X. Image super-resolution using a dilated convolutional neural network. Neurocomputing, 275: 1219-1230, 2018. doi:https://doi.org/10.1016/j.neucom.2017.09.062.https://www.sciencedirect.com/science/article/pii/S0925231217315813

[31] Yu, F. and Koltun, V. Multi-scale context aggregation by dilated convolutions. 2015. doi:10.48550/ ARXIV.1511.07122. https://arxiv.org/abs/1511.07122

[32] Hosseiny, M., Kooraki, S., Gholamrezanezhad, A., Reddy, S. and Myers, L. Radiology perspective of coronavirus disease 2019 (Covid-19): Lessons from severe acute respiratory syndrome and middle east respiratory syndrome. American Journal of Roentgenology, 214(5): 1078-1082, 2020. doi:10.2214/ajr.20.22969.

[33] Chen, N., Zhou, M., Dong, X., Qu, J., Gong, F., Han, Y. et al. Epidemiological and clinical characteristics of 99 cases of 2019 novel coronavirus pneumonia in Wuhan, China: A descriptive study. The Lancet, 395(10223): 507-513, 2020. doi:10.1016/s0140-6736(20)30211-7.

[34] Dai, Y. and Zhuang, P. Compressed sensing MRI via a multi-scale dilated residual convolution network. 2019. doi:10.48550/ARXIV.1906.05251.https://arxiv.org/abs/1906.05251

[35] Roy, S.S., Sikaria, R. and Susan, A. A deep learning based CNN approach on MRI for Alzheimer's disease detection. Intelligent Decision Technologies, 13(4): 495-505, 2020. doi:10.3233/idt-190005.

[36] Center, N.C. NIH clinical center provides one of the largest publicly available chest X-ray datasets to scientific community. Last access on Jan. 15, 2023. https://nihcc.app.box.com/v/ChestXray-NIHCC

[37] Biswas, R., Vasan, A. and Roy, S.S. Dilated deep neural network for segmentation of retinal blood vessels in fundus images. Iranian Journal of Science and Technology. Transactions of Electrical Engineering, 44(1): 505-518, 2019. doi:10.1007/s40998-019-00213-7.

[38] Arowolo, M.O., Ogundokun, R.O., Misra, S., Agboola, B.D. and Gupta, B. Machine learning-based IoT system for COVID-19 epidemics. Computing, 105(4): 831-847, 2023.

[39] Shorfuzzaman, M. IoT-enabled stacked ensemble of deep neural networks for the diagnosis of COVID-19 using chest CT scans. Computing, 105(4): 887-908, 2023.

[40] Chen, H., Khan, S., Kou, B., Nazir, S., Liu, W. and Hussain, A. A smart machine learning model for the detection of brain hemorrhage diagnosis based internet of things in smart cities. Complexity, 2020: 1-10, 2020.

[41] Park, S.U., Jang, D.J., Kim, D.K. and Choi, C. Key attributes and clusters of the Korean exercise healthcare industry viewed through big data: Comparison before and after the COVID-19 pandemic. Healthcare, 11(15): 2133, 2023, July. MDPI.

[42] Al-Atawi, A.A., Khan, F. and Kim, C.G. Application and challenges of IoT healthcare system in Covid-19. Sensors, 22(19): 7304, 2022.

[43] Singh, R.P., Javaid, M., Haleem, A. and Suman, R. Internet of things (IoT) applications to fight against COVID-19 pandemic. Diabetes & Metabolic Syndrome: Clinical Research & Reviews, 14(4): 521-524, 2020.

[44] Anas, M., Roy, S.S., Srivastava, K.S. and Chakraborty, J. Plant diseases classification using neural network: AlexNet. Deep Learning Applications in Image Analysis, 133-147, 2023. Singapore: Springer Nature Singapore.

[45] Ghoshal, N., Anas, M. and Roy, S.S. Chest X-ray image classification of pneumonia disease using EfficientNet and InceptionV3. Deep Learning Applications in Image Analysis, 173-186, 2023. Singapore: Springer Nature Singapore.

[46] Muhammad, M.Y., Fonkam, M., Thandekkattu, S.G., Rakshit, S. and Vajjhala, N.R. Comparative analysis of bit-parallel string pattern matching algorithms for biological sequences. Operational Research in Engineering Sciences: Theory and Applications, 6(1): 322-331, 2023. Indexed in Scopus. Link: https://oresta.org/article-view/?id=554

[47] Strang, K.D. and Vajjhala, N.R. Mining project failure indicators from big data using machine learning mixed methods. International Journal of Information Technology Project Management (IJITPM), 14(1): 1-24, 2023. DOI: 10.4018/IJITPM.317221. Indexed in SCOPUS, Web of Science Emerging Sources Citation Index (ESCI), INSPEC, DBLP, and UGC-CARE. Link: https://www.igi-global.com/article/mining-project-failure-indicators-from-big-data-using-machine-learning-mixed-methods/317221

[48] Vajjhala, N.R. and Thandekkattu, S.G. Machine learning in small- and medium-sized enterprises knowledge management: An overview of the latest trends. 9th International Conference Computers, Management & Mathematical Sciences (ICCM) 2023. 24th-25th August 2023. North Eastern Regional Institute of Science and Technology (NERIST) India. Proceedings to be published in Springer Proceedings in Mathematics and Sciences (PROMS) indexed in SCOPUS, WoS, and DBLP.

CHAPTER

7

Tensor Decomposition in Genomics

Y-h. Taguchi*
Chuo University, Tokyo, Japan

In this review, we summarized the recent development of the application of tensor decomposition (TD) to genomics. Although TD is the old method, TD has only recently come to be employed in genomics analysis, possibly because there were enough data sets available till recently. We hope that TD can be a promising method in genomics analysis in the future.

1. Introduction

Tensor decomposition [1] has ever been used rarely in genomic science. However, recently it was started to be employed in various subfields in genomics. We would like to review recent progress of the usage of tensor decomposition in genomic science.

A tensor is a natural extension of matrix, $x_{ij} \in \mathbb{R}^{N \times M}$, which is associated with rows and columns and is associated with more than two indices, e.g., $x_{ijk} \in \mathbb{R}^{N \times M \times K}$. For example, when x_{ij} represents gene expression profiles, is and js correspond to genes and samples, respectively. Similarly, x_{ijk} can express gene expression of the ith gene of the jth human subject at the kth tissue. Thus a tensor is more fitted with the representation of more complicated experimental conditions.

Although a tensor is fitted to express complicated experimental conditions, this does not always mean that it can help us to understand the outcomes from experiments, e.g., gene expression profiles. We need to have some ways to decomposed complicated information into a set of fragmented simpler information. In this regard, we consider tensor decomposition (TD) in this article. TD is the name of a set of techniques that express a tensor by the summation of products

*Corresponding author: tag@granular.com

of vectors, matrices and smaller tensors and has numerous variants. Figure 1 shows typical (representative) TDs.

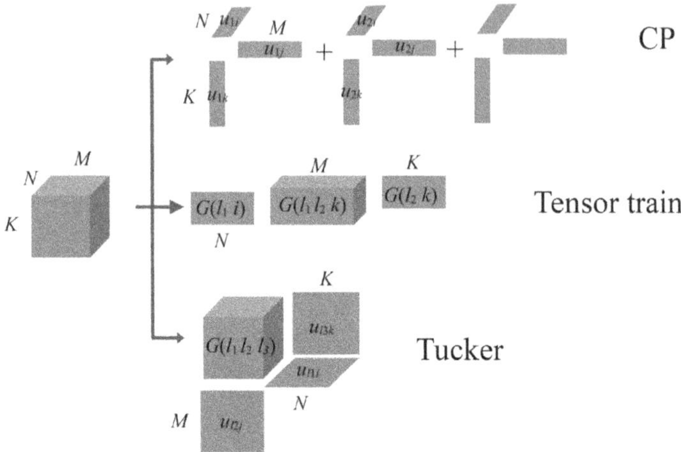

Figure 1. Representative TDs.

The simplest one, CP decomposition,

$$x_{ijk} = \sum_{\ell=1}^{L} \lambda_\ell u_{\ell i}^{(i)} u_{\ell j}^{(j)} u_{\ell k}^{k}, \quad u_{\ell i}^{(i)} \in \mathbb{R}^N, \; u_{\ell j}^{(j)} \in \mathbb{R}^M, \; u_{\ell k}^{(k)} \in \mathbb{R}^K \tag{1}$$

is the most easy-to-understand TD, but has many limitations. All of known algorithm to derive CP decomposition are NP and do not guarantee to obtain the global minimum.

The second popular method, tensor train decomposition,

$$x_{ijk} = \sum_{\ell_1=1}^{R_1} \sum_{\ell_2}^{R_2} G(\ell_1 i) G(\ell_1 \ell_2 j) G(\ell_2 k),$$

$$G(\ell_1 i) \in \mathbb{R}^{R_1 \times N}, \; G(\ell_1 \ell_2 i) \in \mathbb{R}^{R_1 \times R_2 \times M}, \; G(\ell_2 k) \in \mathbb{R}^{R_2 + K} \tag{2}$$

which is frequently used in physical sciences as the name of a tensor network, has superior ability to express the tensor with a lesser number of smaller tensors, but it has limited ability from the application points of view, because it lacks the weight factor, something like λ_ℓ in CP decomposition, to select a limited number of factors; we cannot select a smaller number of features as PCs that have larger contributions in PCA.

The third one, Tucker decomposition,

$$x_{ijk} = \sum_{\ell_1=1}^{N} \sum_{\ell_2=1}^{M} \sum_{\ell_3=1}^{K} G(\ell_1 l_2 \ell_3) u_{\ell_1 i}^{(i)} u_{\ell_2 j}^{(j)} u_{\ell_3 k}^{(k)},$$

$$G(\ell_1\ell_2\ell_3) \in \mathbb{R}^{N \times M \times K},\ u_{\ell_1 i}^{(i)} \in \mathbb{R}^{N \times N},\ u_{\ell_2 j}^{(j)} \in \mathbb{R}^{M \times M},\ u_{\ell_3 k}^{(k)} \in \mathbb{R}^{K \times K} \quad (3)$$

does not have weak points mentioned above, but has a lower ability to get a smaller number of easy-to-understand decomposed components, because it includes all the combinations of $u_{\ell_1 i}^{(i)}$, $u_{\ell_2 j}^{(j)}$ and $u_{\ell_3 k}^{(k)}$.

In the following we introduce how these TDs were used to analyse genomic data set to understand hidden structures behind them.

2. Gene Expression

Gene expression is the primary target of TD [2] although it is usually expressed not as a tensor but as a matrix; when more complicated experimental conditions are used a tensor is a better way to express gene expression profiles, and TD becomes the most useful method to analyze them. For example, Hore et al. [3] applied TD to gene expression profiles to analyze multiple-tissue gene expression experiments. Since gene expression profiles are associated with not only individuals but also tissues, tensors are a more suitable format to represent them. Gene expression profiles are represented as genes × individuals × tissues format, i.e., tensor. In this case, x represents gene expression of the ith gene of jth individual at the kth tissue. Although TD that Hore et al. employed did not exactly correspond to either of the three TDs introduced in the introduction, it is very closed to CP decomposition. Instead of introducing the weight factor λ_ℓ they included the contribution of λ_ℓ into $u_{\ell i}^{(i)}$, $u_{\ell j}^{(j)}$, $u_{\ell k}^{(k)}$, and optimized the following equation

$$x_{ijk} = \sum_{\ell=1}^{L} u_{\ell i}^{(i)} u_{\ell j}^{(j)} u_{\ell k}^{(k)} \quad (4)$$

with a Bayesian work frame. Then they have compared $u_{\ell j}^{(j)}$ attributed to individuals with SNP information to find eQTLs. Ramdhan et al. [4] also employed something similar to those employed by Hore et al., but instead of tissues, they employed various simulations which were called "activities" in their article. Thus a tensor is a format of genes × individuals × activities. Then they have compared obtained latent vectors with GWAS to identify eQTL. Wang et al. [5] also started from gene expression profiles formatted as a tensor of the form genes × individuals × tissues. They have applied something like CP decomposition but with non-negative constraints. They employed GTEx expression profiles and tried to evaluate if obtained latent vectors are coincident with known tissue specificity.

Although one might wonder if gene expression profiles are usually formatted as three way tensors, it is not always a case, for example, [6] also applied TD to tensors generated from the product of matrices that store gene expression profiles,

$$x_{ijk} = x_{ij} x_{ik} \quad (5)$$

where x_{ij} and x_{ik} are gene expression profiles that store gene expressions for the same set of genes with distinct sets of experiments labeled as j and k. It is obvious that this work frame enables us to produce any number, even more than three, of ways of a tensor by taking the product of a larger number of matrices. In this implementation, higher order singular value decomposition was employed (HOSVD) which is one of implementations of Tucker decomposition.

In reality, since gene expression profiles are the most frequently used omics profiles with TD, we can have uncountable number of applications using TD. This section was closed to introduce two recent studies where TD was applied to gene expression. In the above, gene expression must be associated with the same combination of individuals and tissues/activities, since tensor must be genes × individuals × tissues/activities. Nevertheless, I recently proposed the way [7] by which we can apply TD to gene expression profiles without matched samples. In this work frame, individual gene expression profiles are projected as the low dimensional space with the same number of dimensions with singular value decomposition (SVD) and are formatted as a tensor $x_{i\ell k} \in \mathbb{R}^{N \times L \times k}$ where L is the number of low dimensions.

I would like to also emphasize that my method, TD based unsupervised feature extraction (FE) that employed HOSVD, was recently highly improved [8] by optimizing standard deviations to infer Gaussian distribution which is the null hypothesis to select genes. Thus it is promising and can be a de facto standard method for the application of TD to gene expression profiles.

3. Multiomics

The second popular application of TD to genomic data sets is multiomics analysis. Since multiomics analysis is not as popular as other single omics analysis, one might wonder why TD is so frequently applied to multiomics analysis. Nevertheless, since a tensor can represent a bundle of multiple omics profiles as a tensor, applying TD to the obtained tensor is a promising application of TD in genomic analyses.

Durham et al. [9] formatted multiomics profiles as a format of a three way tensor, genomic locations × assay (omics) types × cell types where they employed CP decomposition as TD. They used TD to impute missing values in assay data; imputation is the most frequent usage of TD even outside genomic science [10] and they found that imputation by TD works very well.

I also applied TD based unsupervised FE to multiomics profiles composed of gene expression and histone modification [11] where I have successfully identified genomic regions which are enriched by biological terms related to cancers.

After these pioneering works, many followers applied TD to multiomics data sets. [12] integrated gene expression profiles, methylation and miRNA expression. Methylation is integrated to genes by considering the summation over the region around transcription start sites. miRNA expression is integrated towards its target genes. Then moics profiles are formatted as genes × individuals × three omics.

Then CP decomposition with non-negative value constraint is applied to the generated tensor. The aim of the analysis is to generate the latent variables that can discriminate cancer types. Liu et al. [13, 14] applied Bayesian tensor factorization, which is essentially equivalent to Bayesian CP decomposition without introducing weight factor λ_ℓ, to integrate gene expression, copy number variation, and DNA methylation. The purpose of the analyses was cancer subtyping. Wang et al. [15] applied probabilistic tensor decomposition, named as SCOIT, to single cell multiomics data, which is formatted as a tensor of omics × cells × genes. TD that they have employed did not belong to any of the three TDs introduced in the introduction but

$$x_{ijk} = \sum_{\ell=1}^{L} u_{\ell i}^{(i)} u_{\ell j}^{(j)} u_{\ell k}^{(k)} + a_{ij} b_k + c_{ik} d_j \tag{6}$$

where i, j, k correspond to omics, cells and genes. The obtained UMAP embedding using the obtained latent vectors are more coincident with known clusters than other state-of-art-methods. scLRTD [16] is essentially equivalent to CP decomposition with the regulation using eigen values, λ_ℓ. The targe is single cell measurement and the classification of subtypes. Zhang et al. [17] applied CP decomposition to integrate gene expression methylation and copy number variation. The target of the analyses is survival analysis.

More recently, t-SVD was used to analyse multiomics data set. t-SVD differ from any of the three TDs introduced in the introduction. It is equivalent to CP decomposition in Fourier space. Individual omics profiles are once Fourier transformed. Then CP decomposition is applied to the Fourier transformed tensor and the inverse Fourier transformation is applied to recover the expression in real space. [18] applied t-SVD to integrate gene expression profiles and methylation and identified gene clusters which were further used for survival analysis. [19] also applied t-SVD to integrate gene expression, methylation and copy number variation. They have used the obtained latent vectors to discriminate cancer subtypes.

As can be seen above, most of the papers have been published recently and there are some recent review articles as well [20, 21].

Other than those listed above, I also published many multiomics studies using TD based unsupervised FE. I have applied TD based unsupervised FE to multiomics analysis not including gene expression [22]. I also applied the linear kernel version of TD based unsupervised FE to integrate gene expression, methylarion and proteome [23]. TD based unsupervised FE was also applied to multiomics analysis of single cell measurements to integrate gene expression, methylation and DNA accessibility (ATAC-seq) [24]. TD based unsupervised FE also successfully integrated gene expression, methylation and SNP [25]. mRNA and miRNA expression were also integrated by TD based unsupervised FE [26, 27]. Although TD based unsupervised FE was successfully applied to a wide range of multi omics analyses, it was not widely recognized.

4. Methylation

In contrast to multiomics to which TD was frequently applied, TD was rarely applied to individual omics profiles other than gene expression profiles. Thus, methylatiom is also rarely analyzed by TD. The following are a few examples. Beta Tucker decomposition for DNA methylation data [28] is one of the oldest one. Cell-type-specific resolution epigenetics without the need for cell sorting or single-cell biology was performed [29]. We also applied our method to the methylation profile [30].

5. Histone Modification

Histone modification was also analyzed by TD without other omics profiles. Few examples include the following ones. Epigenomic tensor predicts disease subtypes and reveals constrained tumor evolution [31]. We also performed two studies [32, 33] where histone modificaton was analysed by TD.

6. ATAC-seq

To our knowledge, we are only resarchers who applied TD to ATAC-seq without integration with other omics profiles [34].

7. microRNAs

In contrast to other epigenetic profiles to which less number of studies using TD are available, miRNAs have many TD related studies as follows. The reason is as follows. At first, in contrast to other epigenetic profiles, e.g., methylation, that have more features than that of gene expression, miRNAs definitely have a smaller number of features than that of gene expression. Thus they are easier to treat. Second, since miRNAs are related with many biological features and many studies were published about the relationship between miRNAs and these biological features, it is easy to evaluate outcomes obtained by TD.

Among such studies using miRNAs and TD, miRNAs and disease association was widely studied. Tensor decomposition was used to identify relational constraints for predicting multiple types of microRNA-disease associations [35]. Data Integration Using Tensor Decomposition was performed for the Prediction of miRNA-Disease Associations [36] Multiple Types of Associations Between miRNAs and Diseases were identified Based on Graph Regularized Weighted Tensor Decomposition [37]. miRNA-Disease Associations Prediction Based on Neural Tensor Decomposition was conducted. [38] Multiple types of MicroRNA-disease associations were predicted based on tensor factorization and label propagation [39]. miRCom that employed Tensor Completion Integrating Multi-View Information Deduced the Potential Disease-Related miRNA-miRNA

Pairs [40]. Multi-source Data-Based Deep Tensor Factorization Predicted disease Associated miRNA Combinations [41].

As can be seen above, the usage of TD is concentrated on identifying disease association. Nevertheless, we applied our method to Identify the Universal Nature of Sequence-Nonspecific Off-Target Regulation of mRNA Mediated by MicroRNA Transfection [42]. Thus we have used TD uniquely for miRNAs analyses.

8. Epitranscriptome

All the examples above have studied gene expressions, DNA sequences and epigenetic features, or their combination. Another emerging topic is epitranscriptome, which is a modification of RNAs. Since the expression of RNA itself is regarded to be omics profiles, epitranscriptome has never been regarded as a secondary effect. Nevertheless, since epitranscriptome has started to attract more interest from researchers, it can also be a target of TD analyses. LRTCLS (low-rank tensor completion with Laplacian smoothing) regularization was peoposed for unveiling the post-transcriptional machinery of N6-methylation (m6A)-mediated diseases [43]. Genes' identification associated with altered gene expression and m6A profiles during hypoxia using tensor decomposition based unsupervised feature extraction was also tried [44]. Identification of Transcription Factors, Biological Pathways, and Diseases as Mediated by N6-methyladenosine using Tensor Decomposition-Based Unsupervised Feature Extraction was performed [45].

At present, although the number of conducted trials is limited, since TD can be applicable to epitranscriptome, too, more studies will be published soon.

9. Drug Repositioning and Drug Discovery

Although how genomic data was analysed by TD was discussed in the previous sections, in this section we would like to discuss the purpose of analysis; drug repositioning. As can be seen in the previous section, the purpose of TD is to derive latent vectors which are useful for classification or survival analysis. Nevertheless, there is one topic worth discussing from the point of application; drug repositioning.

Drug repositioning is one of the ways for drug discovery. Drug discovery is usually time consuming and expensive. We have to screen many compounds till we can find promising candidates. Drug repositioning is another way to find effective drugs. Some compounds approved for diseases have already passed other aspects, e.g., safety, drug delivery and so on. Thus, if the known drug is effective to diseases which were not targeted by known drugs, we can reduce the time frame and monetary budget to develop a drug for diseases. This process is called drug repositioning. TD is coincident with drug repositioning.

Suppose that we have gene expression profiles formatted as genes × drugs × human subjects with human subjects composed of patient and healthy control.

If gene expression is that after drug treatment, we can find which drug can make patient gene expression similar to that of healthy control. Such drugs can be good candidates for effective application. Although this is only an example, in this sense TD is a potentially effective tool for drug repositioning.

In spite of this, there are not many studies as yet that make use of TD for drug repositioning. DRIM [46] is this kind of rare case. It does not make use of TD directly, but it applies CP decomposition to integrate gene expression, methylation, mutation and copy number variation and the obtained latent vector is used to screen genes affected by drug treatment. Jamali et al. [47] proposed NTD-DR where nonnegative tensor (CP) decomposition is deployed for drug repositioning. Leggas et al. [48] applied CP decomposition to a tensor of genes × drugs × diseases for drug repositioning. Wang et al. [49] applied tensor of the form of genes × drugs × diseases compiled from the integration of pairwise interaction. [50] applied CP decomposition to a tensor of the form of genes × drugs × diseases. [51] applied CP decomposition to a tensor of the form genes × drugs × cell lines. Iwata et al. [52] also used tensor train decomposition to impute missing values in gene expression profiles where tensors are genes × drugs × cell types. Although it is not directly related to drug repositioning, since it deals with gene expression profiles of drug-treated cell lines, it is indirectly related to drug repositioning.

To our knowledge, we are most extensively applying TD to drug repositioning. At first, we analyzed [53] gene expression profiles of drug treated cancer cell lines, formatted as a tensor of the form genes × drugs × cell lines and identified various promising drug compounds. Then we applied [54] TD to a tensor generated from the product of disease gene expression and drug treated model animal tissue gene expression and identified various promising candidate drugs. We have also applied TD to gene expression of human lung cell lines infected by SARSCoV-2 [55] to identify effective drug candidates. We have also considered [56] mouse tissues infected by SARS-CoV-2 analogous cell lines and identified effective drug candidates. In order to find effective drugs for Alzheimer's disease, we applied TD to the gene expression of a mouse brain during aging [57].

At present, we could not find many studies other than ours where TD was used for drug repositioning. Nevertheless, it will be more popular in the near future.

10. Other Related Topics

The above are all about omics data sets treated by TD. In this section, we discuss more related works.

Avocado et al. [58] employed neural networks instead of linear algebra to decompose tensors. Since a neural network is expected to get more advanced features, when more samples are available, it is promising to employ this kind of architecture. Ikeda et al. [59] applied a tensor of the form of symptoms × time points × human subjects. Thus, it is not an application to a genomic data set at all, but we can integrate this kind of information with an omics data set by TD.

Tsuyuzaki et al. [60] applied TD to brain activity data formatted as a tensor of the form of cells × cells × animals. Thus, it is not again the application of TD to an omics data set, brain activity can be integrated into it with TD in the future. Although there are just a few examples, TD can be potentially applied to any related data sets other than omics data sets. It also might be possible to integrate genomic data with other related data sets.

References

[1] Y-h. Taguchi. Unsupervised Feature Extraction Applied to Bioinformatics: A PCA Based and TD Based Approach. Springer, 2020.

[2] Yuan Luo, Fei Wang and Peter Szolovits. Tensor factorization toward precision medicine. Briefings in Bioinformatics, 18(3): 511-514, 2016.

[3] Victoria Hore, Ana Viñuela, Alfonso Buil, Julian Knight, Mark I McCarthy et al. Tensor decomposition for multiple-tissue gene expression experiments. Nature Genetics, 48(9): 1094-1100, August 2016.

[4] Satesh Ramdhani, Elisa Navarro, Evan Udine, Anastasia G. Efthymiou, Brian M. Schilder et al. Tensor decomposition of stimulated monocyte and macrophage gene expression profiles identifies neurodegenerative disease-specific trans-eqtls. PLOS Genetics, 16(2): 1-23, 2020.

[5] Miaoyan Wang, Jonathan Fischer and Yun S. Song. Three-way clustering of multi-tissue multi-individual gene expression data using semi-nonnegative tensor decomposition. The Annals of Applied Statistics, 13(2): 1103-1127, 2019.

[6] Y-h. Taguchi. Tensor decomposition-based unsupervised feature extraction applied to matrix products for multi-view data processing. PLOS ONE, 12(8): 1-36, 2017.

[7] Y-h. Taguchi and Turki Turki. A tensor decomposition-based integrated analysis applicable to multiple gene expression profiles without sample matching. Scientific Reports, 12(1): 21242, 2022.

[8] Y-h. Taguchi and Turki Turki. Adapted tensor decomposition and PCA based unsupervised feature extraction select more biologically reasonable differentially expressed genes than conventional methods. Scientific Reports, 12(1): 17438, 2022.

[9] Timothy J. Durham, Maxwell W. Libbrecht, Jeffry Howbert J., Jeff Bilmes and William Stafford Noble. PREDICTD PaRallel epigenomics data imputation with cloud-based tensor decomposition. Nature Communications, 9(1): 1402, 2018.

[10] Xinyu Chen, Zhaocheng He and Lijun Sun. A bayesian tensor decomposition approach for spatiotemporal traffic data imputation. Transportation Research Part C: Emerging Technologies, 98: 73-84, 2019.

[11] Y-h. Taguchi. One-class differential expression analysis using tensor decomposition-based unsupervised feature extraction applied to integrated analysis of multiple omics data from 26 lung adenocarcinoma cell lines. *In:* 2017 IEEE 17th International Conference on Bioinformatics and Bioengineering (BIBE), pp. 131-138, 2017.

[12] Inuk Jung, Minsu Kim, Sungmin Rhee, Sangsoo Lim and Sun Kim. MONTI: A multi-omics non-negative tensor decomposition framework for gene-level integrative analysis. Frontiers in Genetics, 12, 2021.

[13] Qian Liu, Bowen Cheng, Yongwon Jin and Pingzhao Hu. Bayesian tensor factorization-drive breast cancer subtyping by integrating multi-omics data. Journal of Biomedical Informatics, 125: 103958, 2022.

[14] Ruo Han Wang, Jianping Wang and Shuai Cheng Li. Probabilistic tensor decomposition extracts better latent embeddings from single-cell multiomic data. Nucleic Acids Research, 51(15): e81–e81, 2023.

[15] Z. Ni, X. Zheng, X. Zheng and X. Zou. scLRTD: A novel low rank tensor decomposition method for imputing missing values in single-cell multi-omics sequencing data. IEEE/ACM Transactions on Computational Biology and Bioinformatics, 19(02): 1144–1153, 2022.

[16] Jasper Zhongyuan Zhang, Wei Xu and Pingzhao Hu. Tightly integrated multiomics-based deep tensor survival model for time-to-event prediction. Bioinformatics, 38(12): 3259–3266, 2022.

[17] X. Gao, Y. Wang, W. Hou, Z. Liu and X. Ma. Multi-view clustering for integration of gene expression and methylation data with tensor decomposition and self-representation learning. IEEE/ACM Transactions on Computational Biology and Bioinformatics, 20(03): 2050–2063, 2023.

[18] Ying-Lian Gao, Qian Qiao, Juan Wang, Sha-Sha Yuan and Jin-Xing Liu. BioSTD: A new tensor multi-view framework via combining tensor decomposition and strong complementarity constraint for analyzing cancer omics data. IEEE Journal of Biomedical and Health Informatics, 1-12, 2023.

[19] Farnoosh Koleini, Paul J. Gemperline and Nasseh Tabrizi. Biomarker discovery in multi-omics datasets using tensor decompositions: A comprehensive review. EPiC Series in Computing, 92: 11–24, 2023.

[20] Laura Cantini, Pooya Zakeri, Celine Hernandez, Aurelien Naldi, Denis Thieffry et al. Benchmarking joint multi-omics dimensionality reduction approaches for the study of cancer. Nature Communications, 12(1): 124, 2021.

[21] Y-h. Taguchi and Turki Turki. Tensor-decomposition based unsupervised feature extraction applied to prostate cancer multiomics data. Genes, 11(12), 2020.

[22] Y-h. Taguchi and Turki Turki. Novel feature selection method via kernel tensor decomposition for improved multi-omics data analysis. BMC Medical Genomics, 15(1): 37, 2022.

[23] Y-h. Taguchi and Turki Turki. Tensor-decomposition-based unsupervised feature extraction in single-cell multiomics data analysis. Genes 12(9), 2021.

[24] Y-h. Taguchi, Shohei Komaki, Yoichi Sutoh, Hideki Ohmomo, Yayoi Otsuka-Yamasaki and Atsushi Shimizu. Integrated analysis of human DNA methylation, gene expression, and genomic variation in imethyl database using kernel tensor decomposition-based unsupervised feature extraction. PLOS ONE, 18(8): 1–24, 2023.

[25] Ka-Lok Ng and Y-h Taguchi. Identification of miRNA signatures for kidney renal clear cell carcinoma using the tensor-decomposition method. Scientific Reports, 10(1): 15149, 2020.

[26] Y-h. Taguchi and Ka-Lok Ng. [Regular paper] Tensor decomposition-based unsupervised feature extraction for integrated analysis of tcga data on microrna expression and promoter methylation of genes in ovarian cancer. *In:* 2018 IEEE 18th International Conference on Bioinformatics and Bioengineering (BIBE), pp. 195-200, 2018.

[27] Aaron Schein, Patrick Flaherty, Mingyuan Zhou, Daniel Sheldon and Hanna M. Wallach. Beta tucker decomposition for DNA methylation data. *In:* Proceedings of the NeurIPS Workshop on Computational Biology, 2016.

[28] Elior Rahmani, Regev Schweiger, Brooke Rhead, Lindsey A. Criswell, Lisa F. Barcellos et al. Cell-type-specific resolution epigenetics without the need for cell sorting or single-cell biology. Nature Communications, 10(1): 3417, 2019.

[29] Y-h. Taguchi and Turki Turki. Principal component analysis and tensor decomposition-based unsupervised feature extraction to select more suitable differentially methylated cytosines: Optimization of standard deviation versus state-of-the-art methods. Genomics, 115(2): 110577, 2023.

[30] Jacob R. Leistico, Priyanka Saini, Christopher R. Futtner, Miroslav Hejna, Yasuhiro Omura et al. Epigenomic tensor predicts disease subtypes and reveals constrained tumor evolution. Cell Reports, 34(13): 108927, 2021.

[31] Y-h. Taguchi and Turki Turki. Unsupervised tensor decomposition-based method to extract candidate transcription factors as histone modification bookmarks in post-mitotic transcriptional reactivation. PLOS ONE, 16(5): 1-20, 2021.

[32] Turki Turki, Sanjiban Sekhar Roy and Y-h. Taguchi. Optimized tensor decomposition and principal component analysis outperforming state-of-the-art methods when analyzing histone modification chromatin immuno-precipitation profiles. Algorithms, 16(9), 2023.

[33] Y.-h. Taguchi and Turki Turki. Tensor decomposition discriminates tissues using scatac-seq. Biochimica et Biophysica Acta (BBA) – General Subjects, 1867(6): 130360, 2023.

[34] Feng Huang, Xiang Yue, Zhankun Xiong, Zhouxin Yu, Shichao Liu and Wen Zhang. Tensor decomposition with relational constraints for predicting multiple types of microRNA-disease associations. Briefings in Bioinformatics, 22(3): bbaa140, 2020.

[35] Jia Wei Luo, Yi Liu, Pei Liu, Zihan Lai and Hao Wu. Data integration using tensor decomposition for the prediction of miRNA-disease associations. IEEE Journal of Biomedical and Health Informatics, 26(5): 2370-2378, 2022.

[36] Dong Ouyang, Rui Miao, Jianjun Wang, Xiaoying Liu, Shengli Xie et al. Predicting multiple types of associations between mirnas and diseases based on graph regularized weighted tensor decomposition. Frontiers in Bioengineering and Biotechnology, 10, 2022.

[37] Yi Liu, Jiawei Luo and Hao Wu. Mirna-disease associations prediction based on neural tensor decomposition. pp. 312-323. *In:* De-Shuang Huang, Kang-Hyun Jo, Jianqiang Li, Valeriya Gribova and Prashan Premaratne (eds.), Intelligent Computing Theories and Application, Cham, 2021. Springer International Publishing.

[38] Na Yu, Zhi-Ping Liu and Rui Gao. Predicting multiple types of microrna-disease associations based on tensor factorization and label propagation. Computers in Biology and Medicine, 146: 105558, 2022.

[39] P. Liu, J. Luo and X. Chen. mircom: Tensor completion integrating multi-view information to deduce the potential disease-related mirna-mirna pairs. IEEE/ACM Transactions on Computational Biology and Bioinformatics, 19(03): 1747–1759, 2022.

[40] Sheng You, Zihan Lai and Jiawei Luo. Multi-source data-based deep tensor factorization for predicting disease-associated mirna combinations. *In:* Intelligent Computing Theories and Application: 18th International Conference, ICIC 2022, Xi'an, China, August 7–11, 2022, Proceedings, Part II, pp. 807-821, Berlin, Heidelberg, 2022. Springer-Verlag.

[41] Y.-h. Taguchi. Tensor decomposition-based unsupervised feature extraction can identify the universal nature of sequence-nonspecific off-target regulation of mRNA mediated by microRNA transfection. Cells, 7(6), 2018.

[42] Jiani Ma, Hui Liu, Yumeng Mao and Lin Zhang. LRTCLS: Low-rank tensor completion with Laplacian smoothing regularization for unveiling the post-transcriptional machinery of N6-methylation (m6A)-mediated diseases. Briefings in Bioinformatics, 23(5): bbac325, 2022.
[43] Sanjiban Sekhar Roy and H Taguchi Y. Identification of genes associated with altered gene expression and m6A profiles during hypoxia using tensor decomposition based unsupervised feature extraction. Scientific Reports, 11(1): 8909, 2021.
[44] Y-h. Taguchi, S. Akila Parvathy Dharshini and M. Michael Gromiha. Identification of transcription factors, biological pathways, and diseases as mediated by n6-methyladenosine using tensor decomposition-based unsupervised feature extraction. Applied Sciences, 11(1), 2021.
[45] Minsik Oh, Sungjoon Park, Sa Lee, Dohoon Lee, Sangsoo Lim et al. DRIM: A web-based system for investigating drug response at the molecular level by condition-specific multi-omics data integration. Frontiers in Genetics, 11, 2020.
[46] Ali Akbar Jamali, Yuting Tan, Anthony Kusalik and Fang-Xiang Wu. Ntddr: Nonnegative tensor decomposition for drug repositioning. PLOS ONE, 17(7): 1–18, 2022.
[47] Dimitri Leggas, Muthu Baskaran, James Ezick and Brendan von Hofe. Filtered tensor construction and decomposition for drug repositioning. *In:* 2021 IEEE High Performance Extreme Computing Conference (HPEC), pp. 1-7, 2021.
[48] Ran Wang, Shuai Li, Lixin Cheng, Man Hon Wong and Kwong Sak Leung. Predicting associations among drugs, targets and diseases by tensor decomposition for drug repositioning. BMC Bioinformatics, 20(Suppl 26): 628, 2019.
[49] Yoonbee Kim and Young-Rae Cho. Predicting drug-gene-disease associations by tensor decomposition for network-based computational drug repositioning. Biomedicines, 11(7), 2023.
[50] Aysegul Bumin, Anna Ritz, Donna Slonim, Tamer Kahveci and Kejun Huang. Fit: Fiber-based tensor completion for drug repurposing. *In:* Proceedings of the 13th ACM International Conference on Bioinformatics, Computational Biology and Health Informatics, BCB '22, New York, NY, USA, 2022. Association for Computing Machinery.
[51] Michio Iwata, Hiroaki Mutsumine, Yusuke Nakayama, Naomasa Suita and Yoshihiro Yamanishi. Pathway trajectory analysis with tensor imputation reveals drug-induced single-cell transcriptomic landscape. Nature Computational Science, 2(11): 758–770, 2022.
[52] Y-h. Taguchi. Drug candidate identification based on gene expression of treated cells using tensor decomposition-based unsupervised feature extraction for large-scale data. BMC Bioinformatics, 19(Suppl 13): 388, 2019.
[53] Y-h. Taguchi. Identification of candidate drugs using tensor-decomposition-based unsupervised feature extraction in integrated analysis of gene expression between diseases and DrugMatrix datasets. Scientific Reports, 7(1): 13733, 2017.
[54] Y-h. Taguchi and Turki Turki. A new advanced in silico drug discovery method for novel coronavirus (SARS-CoV-2) with tensor decomposition-based unsupervised feature extraction. PLOS ONE, 15(9): 1–16, 2020.
[55] Y-h. Taguchi and Turki Turki. Application of tensor decomposition to gene expression of infection of mouse hepatitis virus can identify critical human genes and efffective drugs for SARS-CoV-2 infection. IEEE Journal of Selected Topics in Signal Processing, 15(3): 746-758, 2021.

[56] Y-h. Taguchi and Turki Turki. Neurological disorder drug discovery from gene expression with tensor decomposition. Current Pharmaceutical Design, 25(43): 4589–4599, 2020.

[57] Jacob Schreiber, Timothy Durham, Jeffrey Bilmes and William Stafford Noble. Avocado: A multi-scale deep tensor factorization method learns a latent representation of the human epigenome. Genome Biology, 21(1): 81, 2020.

[58] Kei Ikeda, Taka-Aki Nakada, Takahiro Kageyama, Shigeru Tanaka, Naoki Yoshida et al. Detecting time-evolving phenotypic components of adverse reactions against BNT162b2 SARS-CoV-2 vaccine via non-negative tensor factorization. iScience, 25(10): 105237, October 2022.

[59] Koki Tsuyuzaki, Kentaro Yamamoto, Yu Toyoshima, Hirofumi Sato, Manami Kanamori et al. WormTensor: A clustering method for time-series whole-brain activity data from *C. elegans*. BMC Bioinformatics, 24(1): 254, 2023.

CHAPTER

8

IoT, Artificial Intelligence and Cyber Security: The Paradigms Framing the Future of Digital Healthcare

Viraaj Gupta[1] **and B.K. Tripathy**[2*]

[1] School of Computer Science and Engineering, VIT, Vellore - 632014, TN, India

[2] School of Information Technology and Engineering, VIT, Vellore - 632014, TN, India

Much contemporary research pivots around medical and health sciences, with the goal of increasing the average quality and duration of life. Emerging paradigms, like the internet of things (IoT), artificial intelligence (AI), cybersecurity, blockchain and robotics, show massive potential for use in the future of healthcare. Within the domain of IoT, while initial efforts were concentrated towards the design of small, wireless devices, current focus is towards ubiquitous sensing and computing using distributed networks. AI techniques and subdomains, with specific reference to machine learning and deep learning, have captured the interest of both researchers and the general public alike for over a decade now, and with good reason. This computing paradigm focuses on automated extraction insights from patterns embedded in data, leading to easier and more accurate classification, prediction and analytics. Cybersecurity is essential for protecting the dynamic, modern cyber physical infrastructure. This chapter seeks to explore and summarise the current trends, technologies, challenges, risks and opportunities within and at the interface of these emerging paradigms. We conclude our review by proposing an inter-dependent, core triad of the IoT, artificial intelligence and cybersecurity paradigms; attempting to highlight the importance of each of these paradigms, and their interplay, in the realisation of safe, secure, efficient, affordable, and effective digital healthcare systems.

*Corresponding author: tripathybk@vit.ac.in

1. Introduction

The end consumer of any digital healthcare system is a human being. The goal is to prevent, diagnose and treat health issues, improving the overall health and wellbeing of the patient. This naturally raises safety, security, effectivity, reliability and privacy concerns. As seen in Figure 1, the major drivers of the development of next generation healthcare systems include general population aging [1], rising healthcare costs, and a lack of healthcare resources and infrastructure (as compared to the population dependent on them) [1].

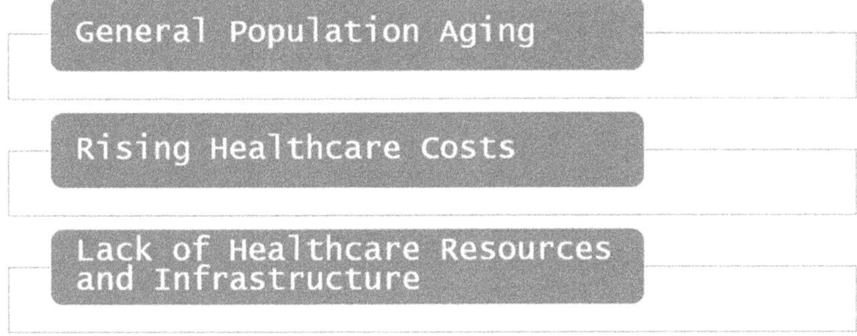

Figure 1. Major drivers of the development of next generation healthcare systems

Key stakeholders in the healthcare system include patients, health professionals and personnel, researchers, investors, data scientists, healthcare institutions (hospitals and clinics, as well as other healthcare facilities), financing institutions, developers of medical products, regulators, and policy makers [3, 4]. The developers of any product or service must recognize the importance of stakeholder interaction, collaboration and adoption to the effective implementation of their product or service [5, 6]. The internet of things, at its core, is a paradigm involving devices connected to each other and to the internet. The design of such a commercially-viable architecture involves sensor design and integration, development of networking technologies and cybersecurity mechanisms, and development of more suitable business models and processes. The three fundamental operations in any IoT network are data collection, and transmission by IoT nodes, and the processing of the received data by the edge devices and the cloud [7]. Today, IoT is still in its infancy; challenges developers encounter primarily are related to infrastructure, interfaces, protocols and standards. The Internet of Medical Things (IoMT) promises real-time monitoring of patients' health by healthcare professionals and institutions, and early detection of health deterioration [7]; which not only improves the patients' chances of recovery but also minimizes the cost of the associated treatments [33]. The true potential of IoMT lies in using technology to rapidly make cuttingedge research affordable, accessible and available to all sections of society [8, 9]. Information sits at the core of practically every industry in the modern knowledge economy. The sheer explosion in the amount of available data puts artificial intelligence at the forefront of this change, due to its ability to derive meaningful and relevant insights from this data. Developers and designers must remember that their customers are already overloaded healthcare professionals, and condensing and presenting the data in a comprehensible manner is essential to maximising benefit from the extracted insights and intelligence [5].

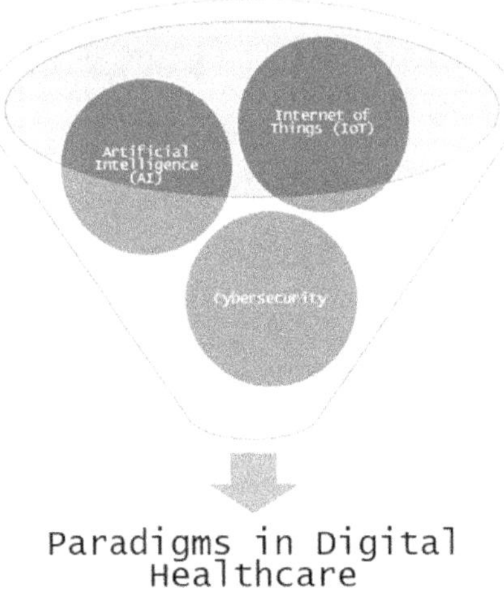

Figure 2. The triad of core paradigms, which are essential in framing the future of digital healthcare

Storing medical records and enabling speedy information retrieval, developing new medical techniques and procedures, continuously monitoring patients, and enabling early diagnosis of diseases are some of the applications of artificial intelligence in healthcare. Additionally, applications of artificial intelligence extend beyond software, extending into hardware and instrumentation, involving error reduction, signal processing, and more [10]. Cybersecurity involves methods, mechanisms and practices to prevent, detect and respond to attacks on cyberphysical infrastructure. The sensitivity inherent in medical data necessitates the use of carefully designed, strict security policies and procedures [11].

Katsaliaki et al. make observations about some key factors associated with the gap in the those who need medical care and those who receive it. They list the patients' inability to recognise symptoms or their willingness to treat their illness on their own as the key driver of the gap. Other factors include situational and financial barriers. Technological advances, creating an Internet of Medical Things (IoMT), have the potential to bridge this gap [9]. Our proposed triad, of IoT, AI and cybersecurity, forms the foundation of such an IoMT network.

2. The Internet of Things (IoT) Paradigm

While sensors and actuators have existed for several decades, the IoT paradigm connects all these devices to the internet, creating an interoperable and interconnected network. Each node in this network typically is portable and lightweight. IoT in healthcare extends from single applications, like the sensing and monitoring of ECG, blood pressure, body temperature, oxygen saturation or glucose, to more complex applications, like wheelchair management, medication management and rehabilitation systems [12]. The objective is to support data-driven decision-making, enhance patient connectivity and increase everyday convenience [13]. These IoT devices can be environmental or agent-specific [8]. The agent-specific devices are wearables (on-body devices), or implantables and ingestibles (in-body devices). A combination of these wearable, implantable and ingestible medical devices (WIIMD) devices hold the key to realisation of an effective IoMT [6, 14, 15]. The time sensitive and life critical nature of medical data, make its collection, transmission, storage and retrieval extremely sensitive tasks [16]. The realisation of effective IoT systems involves two key factors; the availability of, first, energy efficient and cost-effective sensors, and, second, efficient and secure communication protocols [17]. The IoT sensors and actuators connect to form a spatially-distributed wireless sensor network [7, 8, 18]. Advances in semiconductor technology, embedded systems and networking technology are key to the manufacture of IoT devices [12].

A common strategy for building an IoT architecture involves splitting the entire architecture into three layers (Figure 3), namely the device layer, the network/bridge layer and the cloud layer [19]. The device layer includes the sensors, actuators and other modules or devices responsible for the sensing or actuation. By tailoring the signals collected or the locations where they are deployed, sensors in the device layer can be customised to record physical, mental and emotional health data. The network/bridge layer is responsible for

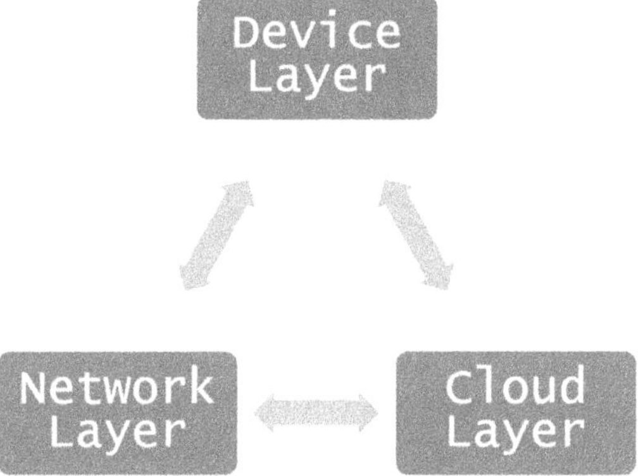

Figure 3. The three layers of the IoT architecture

implementing the appropriate protocols, ensuring secure, efficient and timely transmission of the data between the device and cloud layer [14]. The cloud layer is tasked with the analysis and storage of the data [12]. The sheer volume, velocity and variety of the data associated with an IoMT system necessitate system redesign across the local device-level systems, networking layers and the cloud [1, 15].

Traditional IoT implementations consider the role of the network/bridge layer to be limited to the implementation of protocols [4]. However, the role of this layer, especially in the context of IoMT, extends beyond low-level protocol translation services into higher-level services, including local storage, real-time processing and data mining. Also, a plug-and-play implementation of this layer will, naturally, enhance scalability, reliability and reconfigurability, and ease troubleshooting multiple folds. Rahmani et al. claim that this approach provides solutions to challenges related to energy efficiency, scalability and reliability. Being responsible for efficient information sharing, the network layer is the key to effective implementation of any IoMT system [12]. Another potential reason for shifting part of the processing to the network layer revolves around its ability to connect different devices in the network [18]. This uniquely positions the network layer to intelligently manage events and aggregate data for further processing.

Fog computing appears as another viable alternative to the data processing problem [7]. Fog computing is a cloud computing approach, where devices in the IoT system themselves do not perform any (or any major) computation, but rather send the collected data to the intermediary fog devices. Fog devices are compute-capable devices that exist between the resource-constrained IoT nodes and the cloud. They receive data from the IoT nodes and perform initial processing themselves, transmitting data selectively to the cloud for further processing. This reduces the average distance travelled by the packets, minimising latency and increasing privacy.

Intanagonwiwat et al. [20] describe a method of directed diffusion of data, which is a distributed sensing method responsible for coordination. The entire method is based on nodes that are capable of sensing, computation and wireless networking. Logical organisation in this system is based on a key-value pair system. The benefit in using this methodology lies in its potential for handling large scale, dynamically changing networks. This aids in reconfigurability, and enables remote deployment and maintenance. These networks use short-range node-to-node hops for communication, performing some computation at each hop, conserving energy and transmitting only requisite information to the end-user.

Conventional IoT devices have relied on time interval as a crucial parameter in ensuring energy efficiency during their transmission process [19]. Medical devices often require continuous, real-time requirements and can have substantial energy demands. A potential approach can involve energy harvesting from the environment, including solar, electromagnetic and thermal energy, though such systems will require considerable technological development and a fundamental shift in the current approaches used to design such devices [12].

IoT protocols require interoperability at the device, protocol and data level [21]. Low-cost, portable testing environments can be created on chips, using a combination of physical, optical, visual, chemical and biological sensors [12]. A multimodal sensor approach is vital to high quality, feature-rich healthcare data collection [9]. The heterogeneity in the data collected, particularly in a distributed, multimodal sensor environment, will require careful definition and implementation of specific data sharing protocols [22].

Xu et al. [23] propose using an approach to enhance the accessibility of IoMT systems, enabling real-time access to big data in heterogenous formats. They propose an XML-based, web-accessible metadata model. This model is a three-layered data structure with the layers – value, annotation and semantic explanation. The semantic data model, responsible for efficient storage and interpretation of the data, is supported by a resource-based data accessing method, tasked with the acquisition and analysis of the data.

Another key aspect to consider is the sensor density, especially in whole-body area networks, where many sensors are deployed in a small region [23]. The network implementation will require some modification, in order to intelligently assist in adaptive learning and decision making. The transmission of data in such IoMT systems will be done via the most desired channel, usually, the shortest possible or most well-maintained path. This will require modification of the medium access control (MAC) layer, using wireless channel condition inference. In the Q-value prototype used has a function that is defined to prioritise low channel collision [18].

The critical and sensitive nature of IoMT make the Quality of Service (QoS) requirements of such a system more stringent than that of a non-medical purpose IoT system. A key challenge in quality assurance arises when the need for continuous service uptime and reliability must be balanced by the need for automatic node discovery and mapping within the network. Careful analysis reveals that while both the abovementioned tasks are critical to the reliability of the IoMT system, the former represents the immediate needs, while the latter represents the long-term requirements needed to ensure QoS [7]. Another key aspect of reliability involves considering the variation in demand for certain specialised tools and instruments, enabling institutions to share their infrastructure. This will require the network layer to provision for both wireless sensor and actuator networks (WSANs) as well as ad hoc networking.

The CodeBlue architecture, developed at Harvard University, involves sensors collecting health data, and transmitting them to local health record databases, using the adaptive demand-driven multicast routing (ADMR) approach [20]. Routing is assisted using a path cost table that exists at each node [25, 29]. The best/optimal paths are continuously maintained, accounting for dynamic node movement in this digital healthcare system. ADMR works on an advertisement-ubscription model, where a node advertising a certain data message sends the data to all the subscribing nodes, where the other nodes behave like forwarders, assisting in data transfer.

Khazbak et al. propose a unified mobile-based platform, CellCheck, that provides services ranging from remote patient monitoring and drug control, to health financing and education. They consider using smartphones to make cost-effective, quality healthcare more accessible, and solve the problem created by the acute shortage of medical infrastructure and qualified healthcare personnel. Their prototype involves using a fog-based data transfer layer. Here, the wireless interface selection algorithm (WISA) optimally chooses a wireless interface subject to data size, QoS, and more constraints.

The energy constraints faced by sensors, especially implantable and ingestible ones, is another major constraint in the implementation of an IoMT network [30]. Data transmission emerges as one of the most power-consuming applications of the individual IoMT devices. Wu et al. suggest a mechanism for subcutaneous solar energy harvesting. They study patterns in both natural sunlight and artificial light, varying the location of the solar panel, time of day, weather of the day and the subject's motion. Roudneshin et al. [36] propose harvesting energy from human motion with coulomb force parametric generators. Ye et al. [34] suggest using wireless power transfer systems, which transmit energy for charging implantable and wearable devices, and assist in maintenance and quality checks of these devices, serving a dual purpose.

The resource-constrained IoMT environment requires careful analysis of the memory, compute and network characteristics [38]. The speed, efficiency and energy consumption of any IoMT device is largely influenced by its processor, making the processor's microarchitecture foundational to the device's memory and compute characteristics. The HERMIT microarchitecture benchmark suite, proposed by Limaye et al., recognises the opportunities inherent in the application of IoT for medical applications, but also takes cognizance of the challenges, and risks that lie in the implementation of such an IoMT network [39].

3. The Artificial Intelligence (AI) Paradigm

The sheer volume of data produced by IoT devices creates a data handling and processing problem, which makes AI the prime candidate for the extraction of insights and intelligence from the collected data. AI-based approaches are more suitable and relevant for large-scale autonomous medical systems, as they can take into consideration diverse patient segments, including high-risk patient groups and under-served segments. The primary objective achieved by combining the IoT and AI paradigms, is the creation of a complete picture of the patient's medical profile. This is done by taking into consideration traditional medical data, like heart rate or blood pressure, along with other relevant data, like lifestyle, food and beverage consumption patterns [1]. Artificial intelligence can also play a pivotal role in enabling rapid access to medical and technical research [5]. The vast amounts of research being done makes information overload a likely reality for practitioners, which can work to the detriment of the patient. AI tools can be used to curate lists with relevant information for consumption by healthcare professionals.

In the last few years, there has been an increase in the data volume used and made publicly available. Multiple frameworks for data handling, management, sharing and enhancing cross-platform interoperability have been designed and implemented. In [11], Gupta et al. recognise a drawback of this velocity in research, where they claim rapid model implementation hinders the full extraction, analysis and utilisation of collected data and insights, which ultimately hurts future models. Another trend they note is the use of larger datasets with reduced heterogenicity in studied sample populations, and the methods of data measurement. An increased dataset size reduces the net influence any single record has on the model, increasing the accuracy of the insights captured by the models. However, one must always remember that while the reduced heterogenicity in the studied sample population may reduce negative data records, this can potentially risk the model becoming overfitted or specific to that population. Another point to note is that while the reduced heterogenicity in data measurement methods can be considered a sound scientific practice, AI techniques are capable of analysing such data, extracting insights that benefit not just the masses but also high-risk patient groups. Furthermore, AI techniques can also be deployed to normalise data across different IoT devices, ensuring data coherence and consistency.

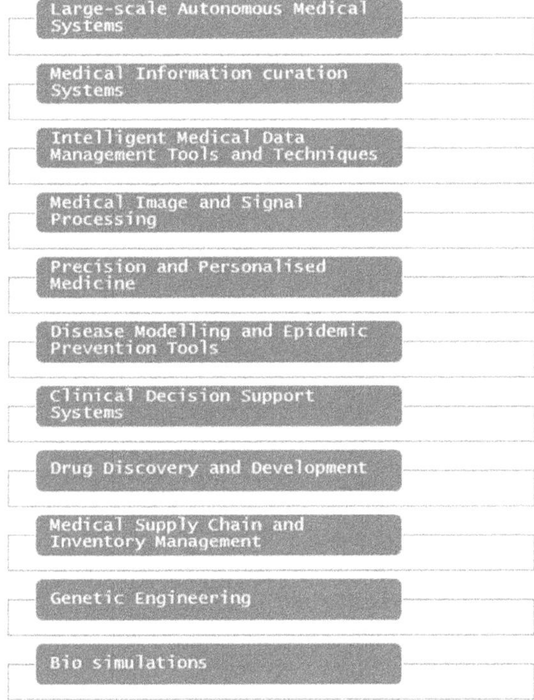

Figure 4. Some applications of AI in healthcare

The effective realisation of this paradigm is dependent on both software and hardware. Multiprocessing and parallelised architectures are crucial to the effective processing and management of large volumes of data. Application-specific AI workflows at both, the hardware and software level, can optimize and accelerate the analysis process. Data mining workflows, for example, can be embedded on the hardware to accelerate the feedback process, both in terms of speed and relative proximity to the patient [12]. Intanagonwiwat et al. suggest using a low-power ASIC to offload basic computing functions and invoke the main processor, when an appropriate workload arises [19].

An IoMT network often records the same type of physical data from a specific individual or group of individuals. Multiple nodes can be used to collect data related to the same or different physical parameters. Data fusion is essential to our ability to comprehend the collected data and extract actionable insights from it. It involves automatic or semi-automatic mapping of data from different sources into a single, consolidated database. Such insights can be gained at both the individual level as well as the sample/population level [12].

The biological signals recorded by IoT devices are prone to disturbances, interference and noise. Artificial intelligence is also a key aspect of efficient signal processing, noise filtering and feature extraction [12]. The application of AI-based image processing and pattern recognition techniques can help identify disease biomarkers, even while the diseases are developing. This need is compounded by the dearth of health professionals in certain specialised domains or in certain regions. The use of natural language processing (NLP) techniques and algorithms can help bridge language barriers in patient-doctor communication and access to medical literature, and can aid in summarisation and contextualisation of information for efficient medical decision making [5]. The applications of NLP extend from simpler tasks, including taking clinical notes or generating a visit summary, to more complex ones related to clinical decision making, data fusion, among others [9]. Healthcare big data analytics extends beyond just analysing health records, including imaging, pathological or genomic data, into other forms of data, like healthcare payments-related data and prescriptions [5]. Analysis of this data holds potential in improving health outcomes and reducing their associated costs.

Most of the data collected is unstructured and does not adhere to any specific pre-defined model. The sheer volume, variety, and velocity of this data, clearly render traditional data processing and analysis methods moot, paving the way for AI-powered, optimized solutions [5]. Precision medicine and personalisation of medical care require a huge volume of data, containing diverse records, from which insights can be extracted and models can be trained. Another challenge posed by the volume of the healthcare data and the sensitivity associated with that data, is the way in which this big data is stored and processed. This creates problems for the realisation of precision and personalised healthcare. Covid-19 related big data analysis, modelling and simulation techniques highlight the potential for artificial intelligence in both individual healthcare treatment, and epidemic prevention and control [11]. Modelling the spread of the disease can help devise ways to prevent and contain outbreaks. Mapping and predicting disease spread, and modelling their stress on medical infrastructure and supply chains over time are made possible using artificial intelligence [5]. Applications of artificial intelligence and predictive analytics extend to clinical decision support systems, drug discovery and development processes, medical supply chains and inventory management systems, operating room demand forecasting, bio-related simulations, genetic engineering, medical signal and image processing, personalised medicine, to name a few [5, 9, 14].

Another facet associated with the use of artificial intelligence in healthcare is the molecular basis of life, where the molecular behaviour of genes, proteins, and other chemical and biological molecules, and their interactions is being studied. [11]. The sheer number of variations in the behaviour of some of these entities, and the even larger number of permutations and combinations that exist in their interactions, create problems that cannot be handled by the current computational hardware without the use of artificial intelligence [11]. Artificial intelligence provides the required tools for conducting efficient, resource-optimized study of these phenomena. Javed et al. propose a machine learning-based framework called the collaborative shared healthcare plan framework (CSHCP). This framework feeds fitness and exercise-related data, location data, mobile usage data and data from sensors to a machine learning model, which, in turn, analyses the data to suggest optimal healthcare plans.

Liu et al. [24] propose a hybrid privacy-preserving clinical decision support system (HPCS) in fog-cloud computing. They employ lightweight data mining methods on fog servers for realtime patient health monitoring, sending the abnormal readings detected for further processing to the cloud. This framework balances the requirement of high-accuracy classification with the need for real-time processing. Data is collected from the medical sensing instruments, and normalised, encrypted and transmitted to the fog server for processing. Then, the fog server either processes the received data locally using a lightweight, single-layer neural network or transmits the data to the cloud for high accuracy processing using more complex data mining techniques, including multiple-layer neural networks. Balancing the approaches used in the handling of big data with the need for data security, Manogaran et al. [40] propose a dual subarchitecture-based system, namely the meta fog-reduction (MF-R) architecture and the grouping and choosing (GC) architecture. The MF-R architecture is a three-phased architecture, with phases for data collection, data transfer and big data storage. The GC architecture groups data into sensitive, critical and normal focus categories, enhancing security services between the fog and cloud computing layers [40].

4. The Cybersecurity Paradigm

Healthcare data records are highly sensitive and confidential in nature, and are protected by ethical and legal codes of confidentiality. Secure storage, processing and transmission of the data is vital to any effective IoMT [8]. Cybersecurity involves the design, implementation and development of authorisation and authentication systems, intrusion detection systems, backup and recovery systems and protocols and policies for ensuring the security and reliability of the system. The protection of the devices, and the associated software, both from vulnerabilities arising out of the use of out-dated software and deliberate tampering, is one of the first lines of defence for any IoMT system. However, one must remember that compromise can occur at the user, hardware, software or network level [13]. Woo et al. recognize the potential for system failure in IoT devices in a network, which are geographically distributed and rarely maintained. Hardware malfunctioning, power fluctuations and outages can also weaken the system (either immediately or over time), which can lead to the services being disrupted. They also highlight the increased probability of fault occurrence in large scale IoT systems. Confidentiality of healthcare data is key to the privacy, security and dignity of patients, their families, and the medical professionals and institutions involved [41]. Man in the middle and tampering attacks can disrupt a system's services and deteriorate its efficiency and reliability, which in the case of a healthcare system can be particularly fatal. Forgery and impersonation may directly compromise the confidentiality and integrity of the data. Such attempts may also bottleneck the system, affecting its availability [3].

While confidentiality, integrity and availability of data are key pillars of every cybersecurityrelated service or platform, health data has additional constraints of data freshness and forward security associated with it. Data freshness requires data to be received in a timely fashion to ensure that relevant insights can be gained in time in order to take the necessary proactive measures. Medical data is connected in a time series, such that the data at one instance is linked to the data at the next moment. Forward security ensures that compromise of a current instance of a medical record does not compromise previously transmitted medical records. Additionally, IoT networks impose mutual authentication and authorization requirements on the system, both at the user level and device-to-device level [1]. The importance of approaches and their availability take a whole new meaning in the context of mobile, resource-constrained IoT devices, where memory, network bandwidth and processing power are very limited. A DoS/DDoS attack, for example, can have severe consequences to such an IoMT system. Traditional networks rely on stationary, non-resource constrained devices. For IoMT, reliability is software, hardware and protocol dependent [25]. Using spam to broadcast redundant or fake data over a network, or jamming techniques to throttle the network, both overload the system's resources, threatening data availability and freshness. Security constraints also arise due to the resource-constrained architecture of such digital healthcare systems [3]. Computational, memory, network and energy constraints limit the complexity of the security algorithms and protocols that can be implemented. By extension, the mobility, dynamic and automatic reconfigurability, and scalability of an IoMT system becomes a difficult task. The difficulty arises due to dynamic network topology reconfiguration, failure management needs, and handling device multiplicity (in terms of computational, memory, network and energy capabilities) in a resource-constrained environment [13].

Authorisation and authentication need to be done in real-time in order to ensure the data can be recorded, transmitted, stored, processed and analysed in a timely manner. Informed consent, which is an integral principle and guideline of healthcare, must be considered when implementing protocols to perform authentication and authorisation. The on-demand availability of medical records and analyses can be life-saving in emergency situations [1]. The abovementioned protocols can make provision for access of such data by first responders, and licensed medical personnel, in case of medical emergencies. An additional aspect of consent involves education, where the patients and their families, are provided with the required information to 'inform' their decisions. In [26], Yang et al. propose a self-adaptive two-fold access control mechanism to make provision for both normal and emergency situations. They propose an attribute-key mechanism for data access in ordinary situations and a passwordbased break-glass access mechanism for emergency situations. Both these systems can have different security policies, creating potential for variation in the access control system, while adding resilience to the system. They recognise the risk of malicious data access in the breakglass mechanism and aim to work towards making the mechanism manageable and accountable.

Another facet in this cybersecurity discussion in the IoMT context is the impact of the cybersecurity algorithms and their implementations on the ability of the system to process the data in real-time. Sarosh et al. [27] recognize that many cybersecurity algorithms are not suitable for real-time healthcare processing applications. They suggest a medical-image focused cybersecurity framework, called logistic regulated quadratic map (LRQ) and logistic regulated quadratic map (QRQ). Both LRQ and QRQ are novel 2D chaotic maps, with compound chaotic properties and a large chaotic range. This technique is particularly important in modern digital healthcare systems due to their use of medical imaging technologies, like CT, MRI, bone X-Ray scans, among others. Resiliency, fault tolerance and selfhealing are also crucial cybersecurity challenges that must be considered while designing and implementing an IoMT system. Resiliency revolves around the aspect that failure at one node does not cause failure at other nodes. Fault tolerance involves security systems being active even in the presence of device compromise, glitches or failure. Self-healing is of particular importance considering the small size, remote deployment locations and resourceconstrained nature of devices in an IoMT network [13]. The data collection approach in an IoMT network involves the collection of data from the sensors, along with metadata, including location, time and the type of value the data represents. The consolidation and storage of this collected information, in the associated healthcare system, can be a potential approach to check for inconsistencies and errors. In [15], Zovko et al. state a mechanism similar to that used in forest fire monitoring systems, extending that approach to digital healthcare systems.

Furthermore, another potential benefit of the IoMT system is in its potential for knowledge sharing, across domains, institutions and geographies. This requires data to be shared via publicly accessible infrastructure, which may involve the packets passing through compromised nodes [26]. Here, the security policy must be designed and implemented to ensure the confidentiality, integrity and availability of data. Growing privacy concerns have fuelled research in fields, such as privacy-preserving machine learning, decentralised processing, edge computing, federated learning, to name a few. In the HPCS framework, Liu et al. [23] implement a privacy-preserving piecewise polynomial calculation protocol that enables the use of a cloud-based multilayer neural network to apply any requisite activation functions to the data being processed. This framework delivers health predictions while preventing data leakage. Real-time processing features like iterative calculation support, which involves reducing the size of plaintext from an old ciphertext to a new ciphertext whenever the size of plaintext reaches its upper-bound, are implemented to blend security and efficiency into the foundational philosophy of the framework. Additionally, the encryption methodology employed enables the patients to securely store their data in the cloud [28].

Gehlot et al. propose a method for ensuring data security and privacy on resource-constrained IoT devices [42]. Deep learning (DL) has been effective in medical image classification, [32, 37, 53] for example, in studying and detecting cancer. During the period of recent pandemic, deep learning was particularly useful in social distance monitoring and mask identification [50]. Mental health conditions could be predicted by using these techniques. Specific applications have been found in brain MRI segmentation [51, 52]. These techniques require large amounts of data, which IoMT systems produce [35]. This makes them extremely suitable for data processing in such systems. However, high energy consumption and data leaks make it extremely difficult to implement deep learning in IoMT systems. Recognising the need for shifting at least some processing to local devices, instead of the cloud, Gehlot et al. suggest using a hybrid encryption method. This method combines both symmetric and asymmetric encryption methods to enhance the overall security of the healthcare data, making deep learning possible, here using LightNet [42].

In Nausheen et al. claim that applications communicating with wearable health gadgets, and the networking capabilities of those devices may be specific targets of malicious entities, as they form unique targets for social engineering-based attacks, and carry sensitive biometric, and health data. The functions, and location of deployment of the IoMT devices may also leave them vulnerable to attacks by adversaries, and/or unintended software vulnerabilities. They propose using code obfuscation techniques to prevent source code reverse engineering, and help conceal APIs used for key function calls. In order to add another layer of security, protecting both the devices, and the processes running on them, they propose using returnoriented security mechanisms, and code Check summing together [43].

5. The Compounding Nature of the Internet of Things – Artificial Intelligence Cybersecurity Trio

The IoT devices are connected to each other, using a wireless body area network (WBAN), [3, 8] and to the internet. The internet of things paradigm builds, and supports the physical infrastructure, where the sensors, and actuators exist, and all the data is collected, stored, transmitted, and processed. The artificial intelligence paradigm processes, and analyzes the data to produce insights, and intelligence to benefit the patient. Clearly, the AI paradigm depends on the IoT paradigm to collect data, and implement any intervention. The cybersecurity paradigm is key to the actual real-world implementation of the two other paradigms, as it is responsible for the protection, security, and defence of patients, their interests, and privacy, intended, and effective implementation of algorithms, and the physical infrastructure that supports this entire system [3]. Challenges related to authentication, and authorisation, user security, privacy and energy consumption limit the real-world implementation of these IoMT systems [8].

Nweke et al. recognise need interdependency between IoT systems, and artificial intelligence. Approaches ranging from classification algorithms and models, and feature recognition techniques to data fusion and predictive analytics, are used to wrangle, store, analyze and visualize the data accumulated throughout nodes in the IoMT system. They also highlight the existence of overlapping and concatenated features, and the limits imposed by using a single machine learning model. In [22], Djelouat et al. propose a compressive sensing-based biometric identification system that uses an individual's electrocardiogram (ECG), reducing energy consumption and enhancing security [8]. Here, the ECG is used both as a biometric mechanism and as the actual signal that needs to be recorded, transmitted and processed [44]. In [45], other biometric-based mechanisms have been proposed by Sun et al., involving gait, photoplethysmography (PPG), behavioural characteristics and more. This clearly shows that the AI paradigm, when combined with the cybersecurity and IoT paradigm, will strengthen this resource-constrained system; and that such systems cannot be implemented without any one of the three abovementioned paradigms.

6. Other Paradigms Foundational to the Future of Healthcare

Interfaces and human-factors engineering are essential to the effectiveness of any digital healthcare system [4, 31]. The front end of the technologies at work, i.e., the IoT sensors and actuators, must be designed to ensure that even patients with no technological experience are able to use these devices. The small size of the nodes and the networked nature of this system may pose challenges related to networking, syncing, device operation, failure prevention, system maintenance, among other functions. Designing semi, or fully, autonomous digital healthcare systems, with natural language interfaces, may be key to deriving maximum benefit from, and realising the full potential of this system.

Cloud computing provides scalable data storage and processing solutions. While there has been considerable growth in processor speeds, the growth in network bandwidth can be considered rather asymmetric; which causes the latter to become a bottleneck in the centralised cloud computing paradigm, resulting in latency. In [3] Arora et al. acknowledge that, "challenges posed in terms of network bandwidth, latencies, reliability challenges, and other security issues caused by explosive growth rate of data, cannot be solved by complete dependence on the CC (cloud computing) model." However, the fog computing approach, which is geographically distributed and works by pooling the local resources together, complements the cloud computing paradigm, attempting to shift at least part of the processing and decision-making to the local environment, instead of the cloud.

Augmented and virtual reality are foundational to emerging methods like remote surgery, telemedicine, visualisation of remotely-monitored patient health data and simulation-based medical training. The cyber-physical-social system, which by itself is not a paradigm, but rather a combination of cybersecurity, IoT and social paradighms [13]. Its importance originates from the fact that the providers of raw data and the consumers of the extracted insights are individuals, who form the social paradigm. The way they perceive a digital healthcare system is an important factor in their adoption, and, by extension, wide-spread acceptance and use of any such system.

MEMS emerges as a potential technology for the implementation of an integrated sensor environment or a lab-on-chip IoMT device. For smaller devices, nanotechnology is another paradigm that holds immense promise [46]. Advances in nanotechnology have the capability, efficiency and flexibility to span the entire spectrum of medical applications, from health monitoring, to smart, targeted drug administration and nanoscale surgeries. In [47], Ali et al. envision a nanonetwork built using two different devices, i.e., nano-devices and nanorouters and two different communication technologies, i.e., molecular and terahertz electromagnetic communication. They note key challenges that arise with respect to device size, resource constraints and communication limitations, and recognise that these challenges must be considered throughout the design process. However, they also highlight the potential in terms of the scale of deployment and the non-invasive nature of treatment.

7. Opportunities

Digital healthcare systems that incorporate the above paradigms can ease patient convenience, and increase the availability of quality medical care across geographies and various sections of society; with the goal here being to shift medical care from the hospital environment to the home environment [1, 2, 12]. The realisation of this systemic shift will necessitate the cooperation of the above mentioned stakeholders, and the convergence of these paradigms, and other systems and technologies. In [30] it is at this convergence where newer problems and challenges, and, thus, newer opportunities arise.

Mobility support, allowing patients to move around in the hospital, at home or in other environments, with the assurance that their health is being continuously monitored, can be game-changing for medical care, especially for rehabilitation [2, 3, 15]. Remote, real-time disease detection and intervention becomes a real possibility in the domain of healthcare [48, 49]. A possible scenario can be that of a cardiologist, who notices a change in the diet, lifestyle or cardiometabolic data, and uses that to analyze the risk of heart disease, and to remotely guide treatment instead of requiring periodic hospital visits [3, 9].

Automated medical prescription adherence monitoring and tailored post-discharge care is made possible with IoMT-based continuous monitoring and AI-powered analyses. Additionally, the patients per doctor ratio can be increased, though this may require current organisational systems, processes and methods to be modified [4]. An added advantage lies in the potential for international collaboration where healthcare professionals and institutions, no longer bound by geographical limitations, can have access to information such as medical data, patient records and healthcare infrastructure providing patients with access to high quality international expertise and facilities at their fingertips. Ambient assisted living technology can also become efficiently implementable with the use of a secure, intelligent IoMT system. Ambient assisted living is a concept that supports elderly people in their day-to-day activities, enabling them to live independently [23]. The internet-based nature of the above mentioned technology will enable uniform accessibility across both the urban and rural landscape.

Relapse prevention, detection and monitoring systems, powered by continuous patient health monitoring, carries massive promise for patients' dealing with issues such as mental illnesses, heart disease and substance abuse. Another application of continuous monitoring is the detection of disease spread; for example, in cases of cancer metastasis, where non-detection or delayeddetection of such malignant spread can be life-threatening, continuous monitoring can prove to be game-changing. In [9] Arora et al. claim there is increased pressure on the medical infrastructure due to chronic diseases, and state that IoT based systems can provide real-time, continuous monitoring and intervention solutions, easing some pressure on the medical infrastructure [2, 3]. Early detection of diseases will also reduce the financial burden associated with medical care, both in the short and long term [5]. The prevalence of chronic diseases and the high cost associated with their treatment create unique market opportunities for low-cost, technology-enabled healthcare solutions. The early detection of deterioration will mitigate risks associated with disease spread and reduce chances of further deterioration [9].

Adverse Drug Reaction detection and damage mitigation is another problem that smart IoMT systems can provide a viable solution for. An adverse drug reaction is a medication-induced injury, that can occur due to mixing of noncompatible drugs or the consumption of a particular drug over a long period of time [3]. Cities, and other population centres, which are densely packed with individuals, are at higher risks for epidemic outbursts. Disease spread modelling in a region, or with respect to a population, will empower governments to prevent outbursts of contagious diseases and contain outbursts when they occur [4]. Prevention campaigns, another vital aspect of public health, which are often left unaddressed due to budget constraints, have a substantial and direct impact on early diagnosis and treatment, and can massively improve chances of speedy and full recovery [15]. IoMT-based, digital healthcare systems also have the potential to aid people in healthcare-related decision making. Interoperability between different digital healthcare system vendors, using some protocols and standards, would also be required. Global interest and investment in smart cities creates opportunities for the integration of healthcare systems with the systems involved in emergency, relief and rescue services and governance [7]. This integrated approach to healthcare and governance may streamline entire healthcare processes, reduce operational inefficiencies and data redundancies, and aid in policy making. A more long-term opportunity may exist in the domain of ambient intelligence, which allows machines to continuously monitor the behaviour and health data of individuals, and deepen our understanding of human health and biology [13]. Apart from healthcare technology, applications for such whole-body area IoT networks can be found in sports management and monitoring systems [22]. Challenges, including human activity identification, health and nutrition monitoring, and personalisation of the experience, taking into consideration factors such as genetics, age and geography must be addressed to effectively realize such sports platforms. Here, a robust, real-time, interconnected and interoperable IoMT system can connect both facets, i.e., healthcare and fitness, providing a more realistic approach to healthier and fitter living [24].

8. Conclusion

The potential benefits promised by digital healthcare solutions, clearly, are built on the backs of the above mentioned emerging paradigms. Of all these paradigms, the internet of things (IoT), artificial intelligence (AI), and cybersecurity together form the core backbone triad powering these solutions. IoMT systems must be developed to handle different varieties, speeds, and latencies of data, ensuring timely, and accurate medical insights can be provided to healthcare practitioners and institutions, and high-quality medical care can be made available to the patients [4]. The compounding nature of these paradigms is evident now, and the work done not only in these fields but at their interfaces will surely increase the overall effectiveness, ease-of-use, safety and security of the system. There are countless healthcarerelated problems faced by different segments of society; hence there lie countless opportunities for the creation of IoMT-based, digital healthcare solutions. Lastly, it is vital to understand that cooperation by and coordination between all stakeholders in the healthcare system is foundational to the implementation of such systems in the real world.

References

[1] Moosavi, S.R., Gia, T.N., Nigussie, E., Rahmani, A.M., Virtanen, S. et al. (2016). End-to-end security scheme for mobility enabled healthcare Internet of Things. Future Generation Computer Systems, 64: 108-124, 2016. ISSN 0167-739X, https://doi.org/10.1016/j.future.2016.02.020.

[2] Leijdekkers, P., Gay, V. and Lawrence, E. Smart Homecare System for Health Telemonitoring. First International Conference on the Digital Society (ICDS'07), Guadeloupe, French Caribbean, 3-3, 2007, doi: 10.1109/ICDS.2007.37.

[3] Arora, D., Gupta, S. & Anpalagan, A. evolution and adoption of next generation IoT-driven health care 4.0 systems. Wireless Pers. Commun., 127: 3533–3613, 2022, https://doi.org/10.1007/s11277-022-09932-3

[4] Bahar Farahani, Farshad Firouzi, Victor Chang, Mustafa Badaroglu, Nicholas Constant and Kunal Mankodiya. Towards fog-driven IoT eHealth: Promises and challenges of IoT in medicine and healthcare. Future Generation Computer Systems, 78(2): 659-676, 2018. ISSN 0167-739X, https://doi.org/10.1016/j.future.2017.04.036.

[5] Dash, S., Shakyawar, S.K., Sharma, M. Big data in healthcare: Management, analysis and future prospects. J. Big Data, 6: 54, 2019. https://doi.org/10.1186/s40537-019-0217-0

[6] Devedžic, G., Koceski, S. and Savic, S.P. A brief overview of enabling technologies for digital medicine and smart healthcare. 2021 10th Mediterranean Conference on Embedded Computing (MECO), Budva, Montenegro, pp. 1-5, 2021, doi:10.1109/MECO52532.2021.9460172.

[7] Li, S., Xu, L.D. & Zhao, S. The internet of things: A survey. Inf. Syst. Front., 17: 243–259, 2015, https://doi.org/10.1007/s10796-014-9492-7

[8] Djelouat, H., Al Disi, M., Amira, A., Bensaali, F., Zhai, X. et al. (2019). Compressive sensing based ECG biometric system. *In:* Arai, K., Kapoor, S., Bhatia, R. (eds.), Intelligent Systems and Applications. IntelliSys 2018. Advances in Intelligent Systems and Computing, vol. 869. Springer, Cham. https://doi.org/10.1007/978-3-030-01057-7_11

[9] Katsaliaki, K. and Kumar, S. The past, present, and future of the healthcare delivery system through digitalization. *In:* IEEE Engineering Management Review, 50(4): 21-33, Dec. 2022, 1 Fourthquarter, doi: 10.1109/EMR.2022.3223112.

[10] Pathinarupothi, R.K., Durga, P. & Rangan, E. Data to diagnosis in global health: A 3P approach. BMC Med. Inform. Decis. Mak., 18: 78, 2018, https://doi.org/10.1186/s12911-0180658-y

[11] Nancy Sanjay Gupta, Pravir Kumar. Perspective of artificial intelligence in healthcare data management: A journey towards precision medicine, Computers in Biology and Medicine, 162: 2023, 107051, ISSN 0010-4825, https://doi.org/10.1016/j.compbiomed.2023.107051.

[12] Rahmani, A.M. et al. Smart e-Health Gateway: Bringing intelligence to Internet-of-Things based ubiquitous healthcare systems. 2015 12th Annual IEEE Consumer Communications and Networking Conference (CCNC), Las Vegas, NV, USA, pp. 826-834, 2015, doi:10.1109/CCNC.2015.7158084.

[13] Islam, S.M.R., Kwak, D., Kabir, M.H., Hossain, M. and Kwak, K.-S. et al. The Internet of Things for health care: A comprehensive survey. *In:* IEEE Access, 3: 678-708, 2015, doi: 10.1109/ACCESS.2015.2437951.

[14] Wan, J., Al-awlaqi, A.A.H., Li, M. et al. Wearable IoT enabled real-time health monitoring system. J. Wireless Com. Network, 298, 2018, https://doi.org/10.1186/s13638-018-1308-x

[15] Kristina Zovko, Ljiljana Šeric, Toni Perkovic, Hrvoje Belani and Petar Šolic. IoT and health monitoring wearable devices as enabling technologies for sustainable enhancement of life quality in smart environments. Journal of Cleaner Production, 413: 2023, 137506, ISSN 0959-6526, https://doi.org/10.1016/j.jclepro.2023.137506.

[16] Alam, M.M., Malik, H., Khan, M.I., Pardy, T., Kussik, A. and Le Moullec, Y. A survey on the roles of communication technologies in IoT-based personalized healthcare applications. *In:* IEEE Access, 6: 36611-36631, 2018, doi: 10.1109/ACCESS.2018.2853148.

[17] Fischer, M., Lim, Y.Y., Lawrence, E. and Ganguli, L.K. ReMoteCare: Health monitoring with streaming video. 2008 7th International Conference on Mobile Business, Barcelona, Spain, pp. 280-286, 2008, doi: 10.1109/ICMB.2008.16.

[18] Ali, R., Qadri, Y., Bin Zikria, Y. et al. Q-learning-enabled channel access in next-generation dense wireless networks for IoT-based eHealth systems. J. Wireless Com. Network, 178, 2019, https://doi.org/10.1186/s13638-019-1498-x

[19] Chalermek Intanagonwiwat, Ramesh Govindan and Deborah Estrin. Directed diffusion: A scalable and robust communication paradigm for sensor networks. *In:* Proceedings of the 6th Annual International Conference on Mobile Computing and Networking (MobiCom '00). Association for Computing Machinery, New York, NY, USA, 56–67, 2000, https://doi.org/10.1145/345910.345920

[20] Xu, L.D., He, W. and Li, S. Internet of Things in industries: A survey. IEEE Transactions on Industrial Informatics, 10(4): 2233-2243, Nov. 2014, doi:10.1109/TII.2014.2300753.

[21] Galinina, O., Mikhaylov, K., Andreev, S. et al. Smart home gateway system over Bluetooth low energy with wireless energy transfer capability. J. Wireless Com. Network, 178, 2015, https://doi.org/10.1186/s13638-015-0393-3

[22] Nweke, H.F., Teh, Y.W., Mujtaba, G. et al. "Multi-sensor fusion based on multiple classifier systems for human activity identification." Hum. Cent. Comput. Inf. Sci. 9: 34, 2019. https://doi.org/10.1186/s13673-019-0194-5

[23] Xu, B., Xu, L.D., Cai, H., Xie, C., Hu, J. and Bu, F. Ubiquitous data accessing method in IoT-based information system for emergency medical services. IEEE Transactions on Industrial Informatics, 10(2): 1578-1586, May 2014, doi: 10.1109/TII.2014.2306382.

[24] Javed, A.R., Sarwar, M.U., Beg, M.O. et al. A collaborative healthcare framework for shared healthcare plan with ambient intelligence. Hum. Cent. Comput. Inf. Sci., 10: 40, 2020. https://doi.org/10.1186/s13673-020-00245-7

[25] Kambourakis, G., Klaoudatou, E. and Gritzalis, S. Securing medical sensor environments: The CodeBlue framework case. The Second International Conference on Availability, Reliability and Security (ARES '07), Vienna, Austria, pp. 637-643, 2007, doi: 10.1109/ARES.2007.135.

[26] Yang Yang, Xianghan Zheng, Wenzhong Guo, Ximeng Liu and Victor Chanq. Privacy-preserving smart IoT-based healthcare big data storage and self-adaptive access control system. Information Sciences, 479: 567-592, 2019. ISSN 0020-0255, https://doi.org/10.1016/j.ins.2018.02.005.

[27] Sarosh, P., Parah, S.A., Malik, B.A., Hijji, M. and Muhammad, K. Real-time medical data security solution for smart healthcare. IEEE Transactions on Industrial Informatics, 2022, doi: 10.1109/TII.2022.3217039.

[28] Ximeng Liu, Robert H. Deng, Yang Yang, Hieu N. Tran, Shangping Zhong. Hybrid privacy preserving clinical decision support system in fog–cloud computing. Future Generation Computer Systems, 78(2): 825-837, 2018, ISSN 0167-739X, https://doi.org/10.1016/j.future.2017.03.018.

[29] Jorjeta G. Jetcheva and David B. Johnson. Adaptive demand-driven multicast routing in multi-hop wireless ad hoc networks. *In:* Proceedings of the 2nd ACM International Symposium on Mobile ad hoc Networking & Computing (MobiHoc '01). Association for Computing Machinery, New York, NY, USA, 33–44, 2001, https://doi.org/10.1145/501422.501423

[30] Khazbak, Y., Izz, M., ElBatt, T., Fahim, A., Guirguis, A. and Youssef, M. Cost-effective data transfer for mobile health care. IEEE Systems Journal, 11(4): 2663-2674, Dec. 2017, doi: 10.1109/JSYST.2016.2533419.

[31] Bose, A., Roy, S.S., Balas, V.E. and Samui, P. Deep Learning for brain computer interfaces. *In:* Balas, V., Roy, S., Sharma, D., Samui, P. (eds.), Handbook of Deep Learning Applications. Smart Innovation, Systems and Technologies, vol. 136, 2019. Springer, Cham. https://doi.org/10.1007/978-3-030-11479-4_15

[32] Bhattacharyya, S., Snasel, V., Hassanian, A.E., Saha, S. and Tripathy, B.K. Deep Learning Research with Engineering Applications, De Gruyter Publications, 2020. ISBN: 3110670909, 9783110670905. DOI: 10.1515/9783110670905.

[33] Tripathy, H.K. and Tripathy, B.K. Applications of IoT to address the solutions for children affected by autism spectrum disorders (ASDs) (Chapter 14), pp. 295-325. *In:* B.K. Tripathy and J. Anuradha (eds.), Internet of Things (IoT): Technologies, Applications, Challenges and Solutions 1st edition. 2017. CRC Publications.

[34] Roudneshin, M., Sayrafian, K. and Aghdam, A.G. Adaptive maximization of the harvested power for wearable or implantable sensors with coulomb force parametric generators. IEEE Internet of Things Journal, doi: 10.1109/JIOT.2023.3269953.

[35] Tripathy, B.K., Parikh, S., Ajay, P. and Magapu, C. Brain MRI segmentation techniques based on CNN and its variants (Chapter 10), pp. 161-182. *In:* J. Chaki (ed.), Brain Tumor MRI Image Segmentation Using Deep Learning Techniques. 2022, Elsevier Publications. DOI: 10.1016/B978-0-323-91171-9.00001-6.

[36] Wu, T., Redouté,J.-M. and Yuce, M.R. A wireless implantable sensor design with subcutaneous energy harvesting for long-term IoT healthcare applications. IEEE Access, 6: 35801-35808, 2018, doi: 10.1109/ACCESS.2018.2851940.

[37] Kaul, D., Raju, H. and Tripathy, B.K. Deep Learning in healthcare. pp. 97-115. *In:* Acharjya, D.P., Mitra, A., Zaman, N. (eds.), Deep Learning in Data Analytics – Recent Techniques, Practices and Applications, Studies in Big Data, vol. 91. 2022. Springer, Cham DOI: 10.1007/978-3-030-75855-4_6

[38] Ye, Z., Yang, M. and Chen, P.-Y. Multi-band parity-time-symmetric wireless power transfer systems for ISM-band bio-implantable applications. IEEE Journal of Electromagnetics, RF and Microwaves in Medicine and Biology, 6(2): 196-203, June 2022, doi: 10.1109/JERM.2021.3120621.

[39] A. Limaye and T. Adegbija. HERMIT: A benchmark suite for the Internet of Medical Things. IEEE Internet of Things Journal, 5(5): 4212-4222, Oct. 2018, doi: 10.1109/JIOT.2018.2849859.

[40] Gunasekaran Manogaran, R. Varatharajan, Daphne Lopez, Priyan Malarvizhi Kumar, Revathi Sundarasekar and Chandu Thota. A new architecture of Internet of Things and big data ecosystem for secured smart healthcare monitoring and alerting system. Future Generation Computer Systems, 82: 375-387, 2018, ISSN 0167-739X, https://doi.org/10.1016/j.future.2017.10.045.

[41] Min Woo Woo, Jong Whi Lee and Kee Hyun Park. A reliable IoT system for personal healthcare devices. Future Generation Computer Systems, 78(2): 626-640, 2018, ISSN 0167-739X, https://doi.org/10.1016/j.future.2017.04.004.

[42] Gehlot, A. and Misra, N. Privacy and security enabling for healthcare data using lightweight deep learning with cryptography. 2022 IEEE 2nd Mysore Sub Section International Conference (MysuruCon), Mysuru, India, pp. 1-6, 2022, doi: 10.1109/MysuruCon55714.2022.9972472.

[43] Nausheen, F. and Begum, S.H. Healthcare IoT: Benefits, vulnerabilities and solutions. 2018 2nd International Conference on Inventive Systems and Control (ICISC), Coimbatore, India, pp. 517-522, 2018, doi: 10.1109/ICISC.2018.8399126.

[44] Steven A. Israel, John M. Irvine, Andrew Cheng, Mark D. Wiederhold and Brenda K. Wiederhold. ECG to identify individuals. Pattern Recognition, 38(1): 133-142, 2005, ISSN 0031-3203, https://doi.org/10.1016/j.patcog.2004.05.014

[45] Sun, Y. and Lo, B. An artificial neural network framework for gait-based biometrics. IEEE Journal of Biomedical and Health Informatics, 23(3): 987-998, May 2019, doi: 10.1109/JBHI.2018.2860780.

[46] Gupta, S. et al. Modeling of on-chip biosensor for the in vivo diagnosis of hypertension in wireless body area networks. IEEE Access, 9: 95072-95082, 2021, doi: 10.1109/ACCESS.2021.3094227.

[47] Ali, N.A. and Abu-Elkheir, M. Internet of nano-things healthcare applications: Requirements, opportunities, and challenges. 2015 IEEE 11th International Conference on Wireless and Mobile Computing, Networking and Communications (WiMob), Abu Dhabi, United Arab Emirates, pp. 9-14, 2015, doi: 10.1109/WiMOB.2015.7347934.

[48] Hussein, A.F., Kumar, N.A., Burbano-Fernandez, M., Ramírez-González, G., Abdulhay, E. and De Albuquerque, V.H.C. An automated remote cloud-based heart rate variability monitoring system. IEEE Access, 6: 77055-77064, 2018, doi: 10.1109/ACCESS.2018.2831209.

[49] Sayeed, M.A. and Shahed, A. iDDS 2.0: An IoT-enabled energy efficient and fast drug delivery system for epilepsy. 2023 IEEE International Conference on Consumer Electronics (ICCE), pp. 1-4, 2023, Las Vegas, NV, USA, doi: 10.1109/ICCE56470.2023.10043376.

[50] Satin Jain, Udit Singhania, Tripathy, B.K., Emad Abouel Nasr, Mohamed K. Aboudaif and Ali K. Kamrani. Deep Learning based Transfer Learning for Classification of Skin Cancer, Sensors (Basel), 21(23): 8142, 2021 Dec 6; doi: 10.3390/s21238142 (IF: 4.35).

[51] Yagna Sai Surya, K., Geetha Rani, T. and Tripathy, B.K. Social distance monitoring and face mask detection using deep learning. *In:* Nayak, J., Behera, H., Naik, B., Vimal, S., Pelusi, D. (eds.), Computational Intelligence in Data Mining. Smart Innovation, Systems and Technologies, vol. 281, 2022, Springer, Singapore. https://doi.org/10.1007/978-981-169447-9_36

[52] Pranchal Sihare, Azeem Ullah Khan, Poritosh Bardhan and Tripathy, B.K. COVID-19 detection using deep learning: A comparative study of segmentation algorithms. pp. 1–10. *In:* A.K. Das et al. (eds.), Proceedings of the 4th International Conference on Computational Intelligence in Pattern Recognition (CIPR), CIPR 2022, LNNS 480.

[53] Adate, A. and Tripathy, B.K. A survey on deep learning methodologies of recent applications. pp. 145-170. *In:* Acharjya, D.P., Mitra A., Zaman N. (eds.), Deep Learning in Data Analytics – Recent Techniques, Practices and Applications, Studies in Big Data, vol. 91, 2022. Springer, Cham. DOI: 10.1007/978-3-030-75855-4_9

CHAPTER

9

Integrating IoT, Analytics and Deep Learning in ECG for Cardiovascular Care

Tuhin Mukherjee*

School of Computer Science Engineering and Information Systems, Vellore Institute of Technology, Vellore, India

This chapter focuses on the ECG (Electrocardiogram) data analysis and explores how Internet of Things (IoT), health analytics and deep learning can revolutionize cardiovascular healthcare. This study investigates various efficient ways in which these technologies are combined. This combination can improve disease detection, personalized treatment plans and ongoing monitoring of any cardiovascular disease. This study, uses ECG data as a primary component, highlights how these technologies have the potential to improve patient care, simplify healthcare delivery, and lower the impact of cardiovascular diseases on people and healthcare systems.

1. Introduction

1.1 Background

Cardiovascular disease (CVD) is a pressing global health concern, accounting for a significant portion of global mortality. Annually CVDs are responsible for 20,517.8 million deaths worldwide according to a report by the World Health Federation (WHF). The economic burden and impact on the health system is in billions [1]. To address this challenge, the healthcare industry is undergoing a paradigm shift towards data-driven approaches. The era of experimental

*Corresponding author: tuhin.mukherjee2022@vitstudent.ac.in

medicine is evolving into focusing on comprehensive data analysis, allowing for a deeper understanding of a disease and the provision of personalised patient care. At the center of this transformation are developments in the Internet of Things (IoT), health analytics, and deep learning.

These advanced technologies collectively empower healthcare providers, researchers, and individuals with highly efficient tools to monitor, diagnose, and treat cardiovascular conditions. This chapter provides information on this transformative landscape, focusing on ECG data as a critical component. It examines how these innovations hold the potential to redefine the field of cardiovascular health, offering early detection, continuous monitoring, and personalized treatment solutions for a large number of patients.

1.2 Significance

The potential which the combination of health analytics, deep learning, and the Internet of Things (IoT) has for the field of cardiac care is significant in the healthcare domain. IoT devices produce real-time health data, which can also accumulate in cloud servers accessible to both the user and the health professional . These devices range from wearable heart rate monitors to implantable cardiac devices. These ECG datasets offer priceless information on heart health.

1. **Early Detection and Personalized Treatment:** The ability of this technological development to save lives through early identification and personalized treatment is among its most alluring features. Healthcare professionals can detect cardiovascular problems early and create one to one treatment regimens by using ECG data and advanced analytics. This is essential for both improving patient outcomes and reducing the heavy burden of cardiovascular illnesses.
2. **Improved Resource Allocation and Cost-Effectiveness:** Moreover, this technological development offers improved cost and resource allocation effectiveness through the use of this data based approach. The health system can use its resources more effectively when it is focused on the areas and treatments that will be appropriate for each patient profile according to their diseases. This ensures that patient care is optimized while also reducing unnecessary expenditure, thereby making healthcare more cost effective.
3. **Reducing the Burden on Healthcare Systems:** One of the main goals is to lower the burden that CVDs place on healthcare systems. Early detection and treatment healthcare systems reduce the burden on hospitals and their staff by minimizing the progression of cardiovascular disorders. The primary aim is to provide more access to patient care and a more sustainable healthcare environment. This is achievable due to availability of uploaded patient data on cloud servers which is accessible to doctors all the time. This eliminates the need to contact patients for data, reducing the burden on healthcare systems.

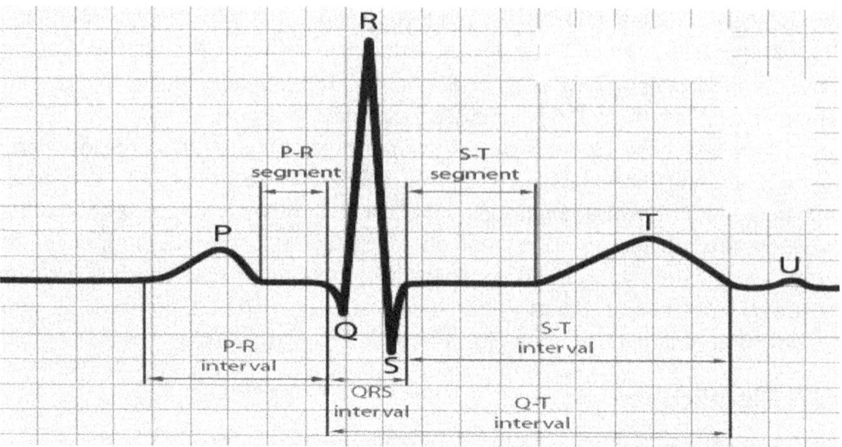

Figure 1. ECG signal analysis

1.3 Description of ECG Signals and Waves

An electrocardiogram (ECG or EKG) signal is an indispensable tool in the field of cardiology, serving as the foundation for evaluating the electrical activity of the heart. This diagnostic model plays an important role in the early detection, diagnosis and ongoing monitoring of various cardiac conditions, making it an essential asset for healthcare professionals. The process of generating an ECG signal involves placing small electrodes on the patient's skin, then recording the complex electrical impulses passing through the heart. In this electrocardiographic device, different components and intervals appear, each contributing to an indepth understanding of the functional state of the heart. In Figure 1, a normal cardiovascular wave and its components are depicted. The P-R segment is the time delay between atrial and ventricular activation. It also serves as a baseline of the ECG curve. The S-T segment represents the interval between ventricular depolarization and repolarization. The P-R interval is the time from the beginning of the P wave to the QRS interval. The QRS interval represents the depolarization of ventricles. It shows the beginning of systole and ventricular contraction. The S-T interval represents the interval between depolarization and repolarization of the ventricles. Q-T interval is the time from QRS interval to the end of T wave.

At the forefront of this electrical activity is the P wave, an important precursor that represents the initial depolarization of the atria. This gentle undulation initiates synchronized contraction of the atria, pushing blood into the ventricles. Next, the QRS complex takes center stage. This complex resembles a peak, symbolizing the forced depolarization of the ventricles and the beginning of their powerful contractions. The ventricles, the heart's power source, are designed to pump oxygen-rich blood throughout the body. Next, the T wave, with its arc, represents the repolarization of the ventricles, similar to the breathing of the heart as it prepares for the next heartbeat. The shape and timing of these waves are important for assessing heart health, as deviations from normal conditions can be a sign of various heart diseases. In addition to these special waveforms, the ECG signal also provides a variety of data in intervals and segments. The PR interval, a subtle pause in the rhythm, measures the time it takes for electrical signals to travel from the atria to the ventricles. It provides insight into the efficiency of conduction through the atrioventricular (AV) node, an essential element in the coordination of heart rhythm. The ST segment, positioned as a bridge between the QRS complex and the T wave, reflects the state of ventricular depolarization, and any deviation here may indicate an underlying ischemic condition, in which the myocardium does not get enough oxygen. In addition, the QT interval, including ventricular depolarization and repolarization, is another important aspect of ECG interpretation. Prolongation of the QT interval may warn of the risk of ventricular arrhythmia. In summary, the ECG signal, with its P waves, QRS complexes, T waves and the wealth of information contained in its intervals and segments, provides a complete picture on which the electrical activity of the heart is expressed.

These signals are essential to healthcare professionals because they aid in the diagnosis and management of a multitude of heart diseases, including arrhythmias, myocardial infarction, and conduction abnormalities. With this effective, and informative tool, the field of cardiology continues to advance in its mission to protect and improve heart health. The integration of ECG devices into 5G networks, combined with cloud databases and bluetooth, represents a transformational advancement in healthcare. It enables high-quality real-time transmission of ECG data, improving remote patient monitoring with the collection of patient data and remote treatment. This combination ensures rapid detection of cardiac abnormalities, supports one-on-one consultations with healthcare professionals, and improves data security with the powerful capabilities of a cloud-based database. 5G's scalability and edge computing reduce latency, ensuring fast access to critical information. Additionally, smooth integration with cloud computing enables advanced data storage and analytics. Rapid, real-time transmission of ECG data during an emergency helps save lives by providing immediate information to healthcare providers. Additionally, this integration drives innovation in ECG technology, paving the way for AI-based analytics and the use of cloud resources for complex calculations. This approach will ultimately enhance the quality of cardiovascular care while improving data access, security, and analysis.

2. Simple Iot and 5G Enabled ECG Model

This model presents an advanced ECG device leveraging 5G, WiFi, Bluetooth, cloud storage and deep learning that smoothly integrates cutting-edge technologies for comprehensive heart monitoring. This device, usually in compact form , connects wirelessly to a tablet or a smartphone. 5G connectivity ensures fast and reliable real-time transmission of high-quality ECG data. This allows immediate access to information about the patient's heart, allowing for rapid intervention and continuous remote monitoring by doctors. The inclusion of WiFi and Bluetooth further enhances connectivity options, providing flexibility and compatibility with a wide range of devices. The ECG device is designed for user-friendly interaction with a tablet or a smartphone. Through a dedicated app, users can initiate ECG measurements, view real-time data, and receive immediate feedback on their heart health. Smooth integration with cloud storage ensures centralized and secure data management. ECG readings are automatically uploaded to the cloud, allowing healthcare professionals and patients to easily access them. The device's compatibility with Bluetooth enables additional features, such as connecting to wearable accessories for continuous monitoring or syncing with health and fitness apps. The collected ECG data is securely stored in the cloud, providing a complete and accessible history of heart activity. In emergency situations or during in-person consultations, healthcare professionals can remotely access real-time ECG data on their tablets or smartphones. Cloud-based storage ensures that historical data is always available for trend analysis, facilitating personalized healthcare planning.

In Figure 2, we can see a portable ECG device which is connected to a smartphone via a dedicated app which shows real-time data on the device. The data which is shown on the smartphone can be instantly uploaded on the cloud server using 5G, WiFi or Bluetooth. This real time data can be easily accessed

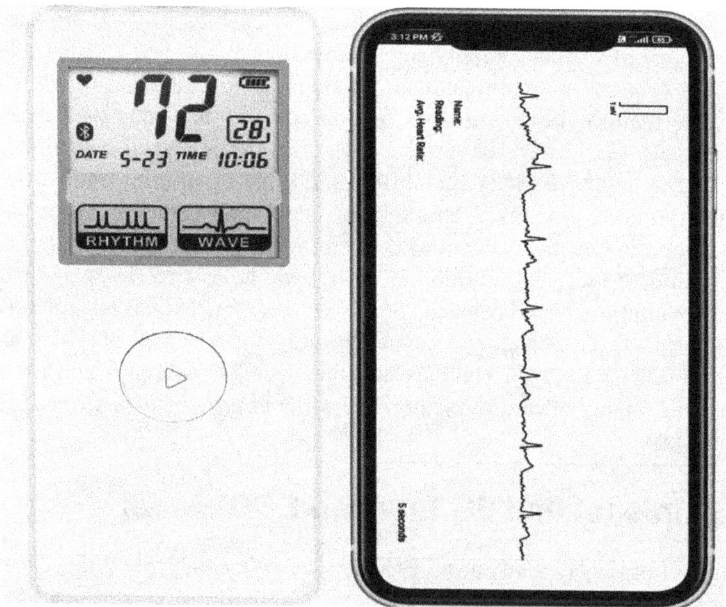

Figure 2. Real time data on user's phone using portable device and dedicated app on smartphone

by the healthcare professional for regular checkups, monitoring or during times of emergency.

An IoT-based ECG system is a complex ecosystem designed to provide comprehensive cardiovascular health monitoring. In Figure 3, the system starts with an ECG sensor, a strategically placed device that captures and converts complex electrical signals emitted from the heart into digital data. This raw data is then processed and managed by a microcontroller, which not only monitors the conversion of analog signals to digital signals but also coordinates the continuous flow of information within the device. The connectivity aspect of the system is supported by a flexible Bluetooth/WiFi module. The Bluetooth function enables short-range wireless communication, establishing a connection between the ECG device and the paired smartphone. At the same time, the WiFi component expands the spectrum, allowing the device to interact with local networks, possibly in the user's home environment. The incorporation of the 5G module in Figure 3 stands out as a key feature, ensuring high-speed data transmission and low latency. This module serves as a gateway that allows the device to connect to remote cloud servers, paving the way for deeper data analysis and processing. The user interface is presented primarily through a dedicated smartphone app(application). This app

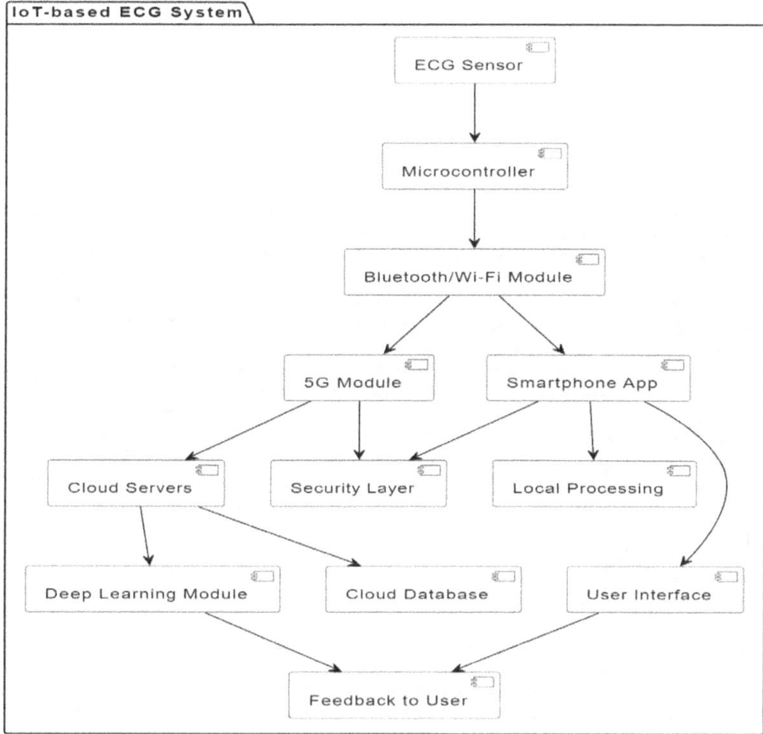

Figure 3. Flowchart on how an Iot based ECG system works and provides real time data to the user

acts as a channel between the user and the ECG device, establishing a Bluetooth connection to support real-time data transmission. The app is integrated with a user-friendly interface that presents live ECG data, providing visual images of the heart's electrical activity. It also acts as a control center, allowing users to start or stop ECG recordings and providing a platform to interact with the entire system. A local processing layer in the smartphone application further refines the raw data before transmitting it to the cloud. This local processing can include basic signal analysis or noise filtering, optimizing sent data for more complex analysis while minimizing bandwidth usage. In Figure 3 we can see the data received going to cloud servers, from cloud servers the data gets uploaded to many cloud databases which can handle various data sets. These databases are easily accessible to doctors in times of emergency or regular check-ups. The app is integrated with a user-friendly interface that presents live ECG data, providing visual images of the heart's electrical activity and feedback.

Cloud servers host deep learning models that analyze ECG data to gain health insights. The smartphone app provides real-time feedback and generates alerts for potential problems. Users can configure settings, view historical data, and share information with medical professionals. A secure cloud database stores data for long-term analysis in compliance with strict privacy protections and health data regulations. This integrated system ensures continuous and easy-to-use heart health monitoring.

In Figure 4 the ECG sensor capturing electrical signals from the heart, which are then processed and digitized by a microcontroller. To support communication, a wireless module, such as WiFi or 5G is provided. Optionally, a local storage

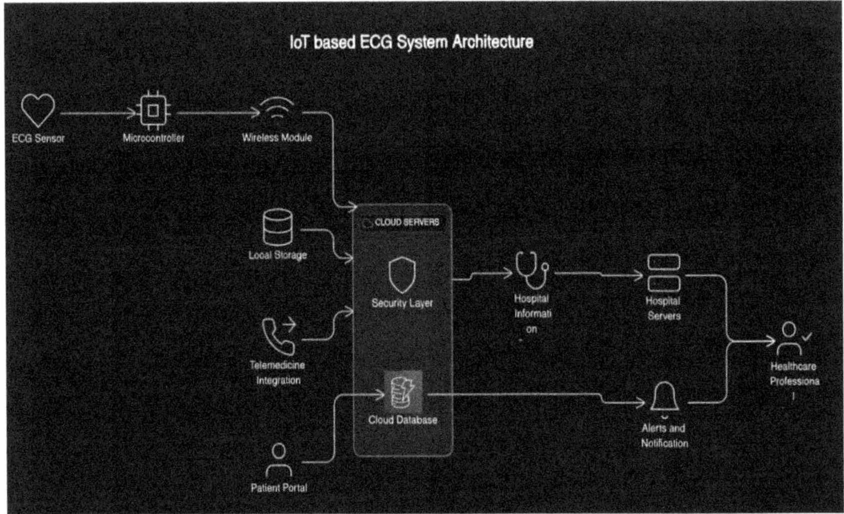

Figure 4. Transfer of real-time data from mobile ECG device to healthcare professional via cloud servers

component temporarily holds ECG data for backup purposes. The data is then transmitted to the cloud server through secure channels, where it finds a secure location in a cloud-based database. Security measures, including encryption and authentication, protect data during transmission and storage. Integration with established hospital information systems, allows for periodic or event-triggered transmission of ECG data from the cloud to hospital servers. Here, data is received, stored and seamlessly integrated into the hospital's electronic health records. Healthcare professionals can access this information through the hospital information system, allowing for remote monitoring and timely medical intervention. Additionally, the system generates alerts for important events and sends notifications to designated personnel for immediate attention. Optional features include patient access to their ECG data through a secure online portal and integration with telemedicine platforms for remote consultations. This architecture ensures efficient data flow, facilitating seamless healthcare monitoring and intervention.

3. Cardiovascular Rhythm Detection by ECG Waves and Signals

3.1 Relation

In this part of the chapter we will see the various cardiovascular rhythms and how ECG detects them by waves and signals.

Heart rate, expressed by interpreting an electrocardiogram (ECG or EKG), serves as a window into the dynamic coordination of heart rhythms. During standard sinus rhythm (SNR), the heart's natural pacemaker triggers a coordinated sequence of events in which the P wave, QRS complex, and T wave unfold subtly on the ECG. In this region, sinus bradycardia appears as an aberration characterized by a slower heart rate, but the ECG retains the familiar pattern, although the beat frequency is reduced. In contrast, sinus tachycardia signals an accelerated rhythm, with the ECG retaining the same recognizable pattern but at an increased frequency. Acute sinus arrhythmia causes abnormalities that are synchronous with normal breathing patterns, while sinus outflow tract obstruction and sinus arrest mean temporary cessation of the normal conduction of electrical signals from the sinus node. Moving deeper into the ECG context, the presence of premature atrial contractions (PACs) disrupt regular rhythms in the context of NSR. Supraventricular tachycardia (SVT) is manifested by rapid atrial and ventricular rhythms, combined on ECG. Atrial fibrillation (AFib) and atrial flutter add complexity, describing irregular atrial rhythms, where AFib describes chaotic ventricular responses and irregular P waves, while atrial flutter produces a distinctive "sawtooth" pattern. The sophistication extends to atrial rhythms, each degree of atrioventricular block (1° AVB, 2° AVB types I and II, 2° AVB 2:1 and 3° AVB Block) junctional rhythms.

Wandering pacemakers introduce different pacemaker sites into the atria, leading to subtle but noticeable changes on the ECG. Venturing into the ventricular domains, premature ventricular contractions (PVCs), spontaneous ventricular rhythms, and ventricular tachycardia (VTach) imprint distinctive patterns on the ECG. Accelerated ventricular rhythm means faster ventricular rhythm, while ventricular fibrillation (VFib) presents as chaotic and life-threatening electrical activity in the ventricles. An in-depth understanding of the different heart rhythms and their associated ECG patterns is paramount for clinicians. This understanding facilitates accurate diagnosis and effective management of a variety of cardiac pathologies, highlighting the central role of the ECG in guiding clinical decisions and optimizing patient care .

3.2 Detection

The process of detecting heart rhythms using an electrocardiogram (ECG) involves a series of complex steps that provide a comprehensive view of the heart's electrical activity (Figure 5). To begin this diagnostic procedure, electrodes are strategically placed on specific areas of the body, usually on the limbs and chest, with the primary goal of picking up electrical signals coming from the heart. These electrodes act as sensors, detecting electrical impulses generated during each phase of the cardiac cycle. The received signals, which are relatively weak at this stage, undergo amplification. Amplification is important because it improves the strength of these signals, making them easier to measure and more distinct from any background noise that might affect the accuracy of the recorded data. After amplification, the signal is carefully processed. This step involves applying filters to remove any unwanted noise or artifacts that may be detected during signal acquisition. The aim here is to ensure that data is recorded as clearly and accurately as possible, thereby providing a reliable basis for further analysis. The processed signals are then represented graphically on paper or an ECG screen. In this visual representation, time is plotted on the horizontal axis, while voltage is plotted on the vertical axis. The resulting graph displays distinct waves that correspond to different phases of the cardiac cycle. Specifically, the P wave represents atrial depolarization, the QRS complex signifies ventricular depolarization, and the T wave indicates ventricular repolarization. Further analysis involves measuring intervals between these waves, such as the PR and QT intervals. Deviations from normal values in these intervals can offer valuable insights into potential cardiac abnormalities. Additionally, the overall rhythm of the heart is assessed by observing the regularity of the waves and examining the relationship between atrial and ventricular activity. This meticulous analysis is the foundation for clinicians in the diagnosis of various cardiac conditions, including arrhythmias, conduction abnormalities, and ischemia. Although detailed written explanations are provided ,there is a The complex relationship between ECG signals and heart rates can be understood by upcoming simulation (Figures 6-9).

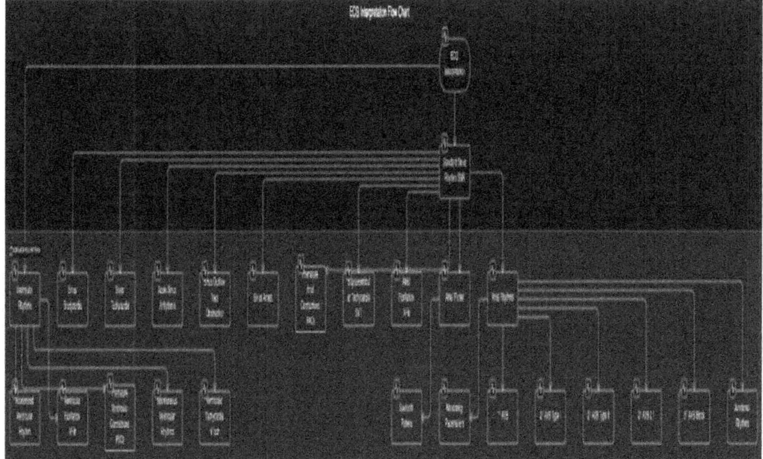

Figure 5. ECG Interpretation of cardiovascular rhythms

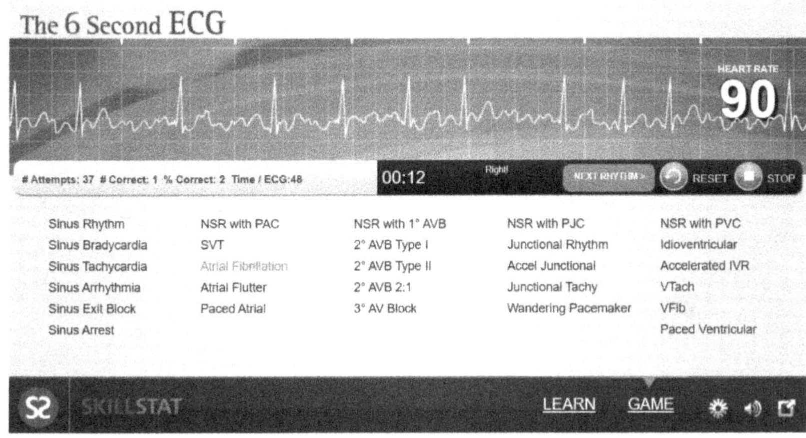

Figure 6. Simulation showing Atrial Fibrillation

3.3 Cardiovascular Rhythms and Simulations

Cardiovascular rhythm simulation plays a significant role in improving our understanding of the complex dynamics of the heart's electrical activities. These simulations involve creating computer models that copy the complex interactions of ion channels, cellular electrophysiology, and tissue conduction in the cardiac system. Using mathematical equations and computer algorithms, these models can reproduce numerous heart rhythms, from normal sinus rhythm to various arrhythmias and abnormalities. By adjusting parameters and incorporating physiological variations, researchers can simulate situations that mimic real-world conditions, allowing for in-depth exploration and analysis.

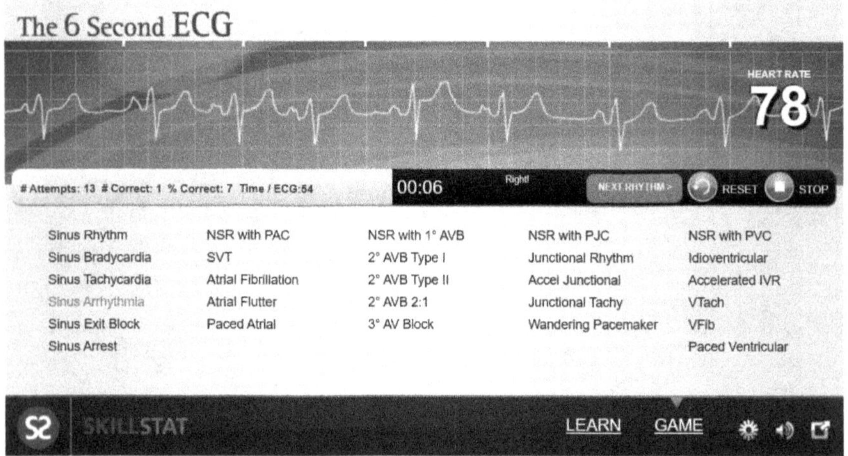

Figure 7. Simulation showing sinus arrhythmia

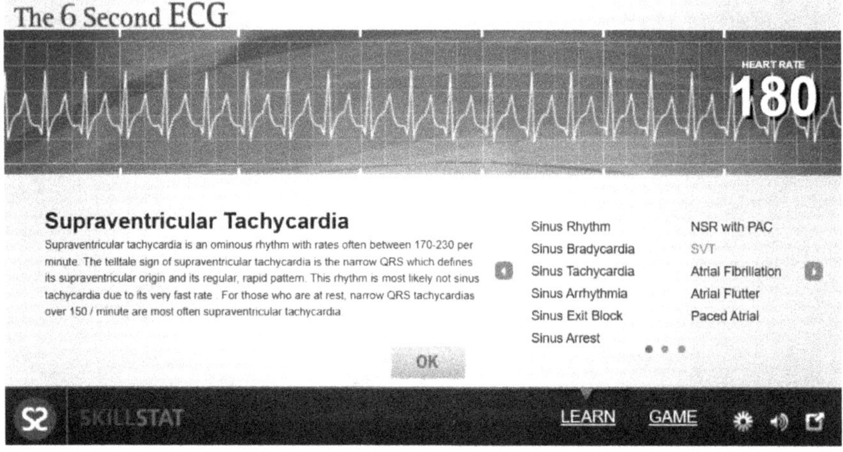

Figure 8. Simulation showing supraventricular tachycardia

These simulations provide valuable information on arrhythmia mechanisms, thus contributing to the development and improvement of diagnostic tools and therapeutic interventions. Additionally, heart rate simulation serves as a testing ground to validate new technologies, such as implantable devices and antiarrhythmic drugs, improving the ability to understand, diagnose, and treat a variety of diseases.

Atrial fibrillation is an irregular and often very rapid heart rhythm as we can see in Figure 6. During atrial fibrillation, the heart's upper chambers called the atria beat chaotically and irregularly. They beat out of sync with the lower heart chambers called ventricles.

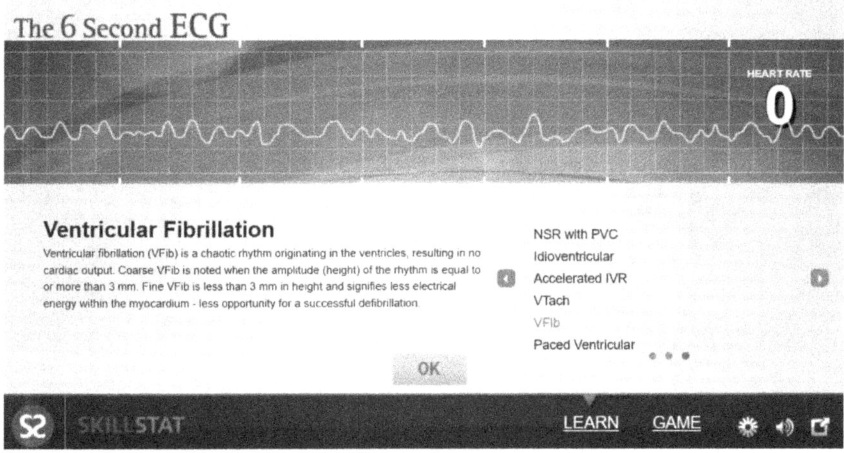

Figure 9. Simulation showing ventricular fibrillation

It is a type of abnormal heart rhythm when the heart beats at a different rate when a person breathes in and breathes out.It can be a changing sinus node rate with the respiratory cycle. In Figure 7 a particular shift in the cardiac rhythm can be observed in the center and at the right end.

In Figure 8 we can see a fast and non sinus heart rate with its explanation.

During ventricular fibrillation the lower heart chambers contract rapidly. As a result the heart doesn't pump blood to the rest of the body. In Figure 9 we can see this exact thing, a chaotic rhythm leading to 0 heart rate. It is the most frequent cause of sudden cardiac death.

4. Prediction: Accuracy in Datasets and Models

The accuracy and efficiency of machine learning models depends heavily on the quality and diversity of the datasets used for training and predictions. These datasets provide the foundation for these models to learn to distinguish complex patterns and make accurate predictions. For optimal performance, a comprehensive and well-organized data set is required, covering a wide range of heart rates including both normal and pathological conditions. The efficiency of the dataset ensures that the model can identify nuances associated with different cardiac conditions, thereby improving its generalization ability. Additionally, the accuracy of machine learning models in ECG interpretation depends on exposure to variations in patient demographics, clinical parameters, and recorded, driving conditions ability to adapt to real world situations. Regularly updating and expanding datasets with new cases and emerging models is paramount to keeping models abreast of developments in heart disease treatments, contributing to continued learning and improvement. The ultimate goal of these machine learning models in the context of ECG analysis is to make

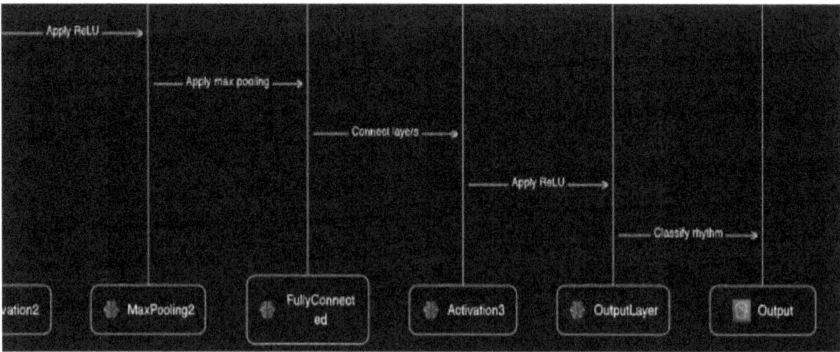

Figure 10: ECG signal processing using CNN

accurate predictions about the presence or absence of specific cardiac conditions based on input data. These predictions, derived from learning during the training phase, have important implications for clinical decision making. Therefore, continuous improvement of datasets and model optimization is essential to maintain and improve prediction accuracy in different clinical settings, thereby ensuring that this machine learning tool has become a valuable asset in the field of cardiovascular health.

4.1 Calculating *t* Values and % Difference

t values are used to calculate the difference between two sample sets generally between a real ECG set and the prototype. This is given by equation (1) below.

$$t = (\overline{x} - \mu)/(s/\sqrt{n}) \tag{1}$$

$\bar{x}$ – sample mean
μ – hypothesized population mean
s – sample standard deviation
n – sample size

Equation of percentage difference is given by:

%difference = mod Expected – Actual/Expected + Actual/2*100%

where Expected is the real ECG set, and Actual is the prototype

5. Utilizing CNN in Classifying ECG Signals

The use of convolutional neural networks (CNN) to classify electrocardiogram (ECG) signals represents an innovative application of deep learning in cardiovascular diagnostics. CNNs, originally designed for image processing, have been adapted to process data such as time series, making them well suited for ECG analysis. In this context, each ECG signal is considered as a one-dimensional image and the CNN architecture is designed to automatically learn and extract relevant and useful features from these representations. The power of CNN lies in its ability to capture local patterns in input data through convolutional layers. These layers apply filters to small segments of the ECG signal, allowing the network to recognize specific timing patterns that can indicate different heart rhythms or abnormalities. Subsequent layers, including pooling layers and fully connected layers, process these learned features, allowing the model to distinguish complex relationships in ECG data. The training process involves presenting the CNN with a labelled dataset of ECG signals, allowing the network to tune its internal parameters to accurately classify different cardiac conditions. Importantly, CNN can automatically learn and extract relevant features from raw ECG data, eliminating the need for manual feature processing. The application of CNN in ECG analysis has shown promise in tasks such as detecting arrhythmias, identifying patterns of ischemia, and classifying various cardiac abnormalities. Once trained, the CNN can be deployed for real-time ECG analysis, providing rapid and automated heart disease diagnosis and classification. However, successful implementation requires ongoing collaboration with healthcare professionals to validate the accuracy and appropriateness of the model in clinical situations.

Algorithm to construct ECG signal processing using CNN

1. **Input (ECG Signal):**
   - This is where the raw ECG signal is fed into the network. Each data point in the ECG signal represents the electrical activity of the heart over time.
2. **Convolutional Layer:**
   - The convolutional layer applies filters to the input ECG signal. These filters capture local patterns or features, allowing the network to identify specific temporal characteristics that are relevant to cardiac rhythms.
3. **Activation (e.g., ReLU - Rectified Linear Unit):**
   - After the convolutional operation, an activation function is applied element-wise to the output. ReLU is a common activation function that introduces non-linearity to the model.
4. **Max Pooling:**
   - Max pooling reduces the spatial dimensions of the data by retaining the maximum value within a certain window. This helps to down-sample the features and focus on the most relevant information.
5. **Fully Connected Layer:**
   - The fully connected layer connects every neuron from the previous layer to every neuron in this layer. This layer integrates the features learned from the convolutional layers.
6. **Activation (e.g., ReLU):**
   - Another activation function is applied to introduce non-linearity.
7. **Output Layer (Cardiac Rhythm Classes):**
   - The final layer produces the output, which represents the predicted classes of cardiac rhythms. Each neuron in this layer corresponds to a specific cardiac rhythm class, and the network predicts the class with the highest activation.

6. Algorithms to Classify Various Heart Diseases

In this chapter we shall not go deep into any particular algorithm, so this shall just be an overview. When it comes to the classification of heart diseases using machine learning algorithms, several approaches can be effective. The choice of algorithm depends on various factors, including the size and quality of the dataset, the specific task or type of heart disease to be classified , and the computational resources available. Here are some commonly used algorithms for heart disease classification:

1. **Logistic Regression:** Logistic regression is a simple and interpretable algorithm that can be effective for binary classification tasks, such as determining whether a patient has a heart disease or not.
2. **Decision Trees:** Decision trees and ensemble methods like Random Forest and Gradient Boosting can be useful for heart disease classification. They can handle both binary and multiclass classification tasks and are interpretable.
3. **Support Vector Machines (SVM):** SVMs are effective for binary classification tasks and can be particularly useful when you have a smaller dataset. They work well in high-dimensional spaces and are good at finding a clear separation margin between classes.
4. **k-Nearest Neighbors (k-NN):** k-NN is a simple algorithm that can work well for classification tasks. It classifies data points based on the majority class among their k-nearest neighbours.
5. **Support Vector Machine with a Radial Basis Function (SVM-RBF):** This is an extension of SVM that can handle non-linear classification tasks effectively by mapping data into a higher-dimensional space using radial basis functions.
6. **Principal Component Analysis (PCA) :** PCA is a dimensionality reduction technique. It can be used in combination with other classification algorithms to reduce the dimensionality of the data and improve the efficiency of the model.
7. **Gradient Boosting:** Algorithms like XGBoost, LightGBM, and CatBoost are popular gradient boosting techniques that are often used for classification tasks. They can handle both binary and multiclass problems and are known for their high performance.

7. Conclusion

In this chapter I have shown the integration of ECG-based care with the developments of IoT, analytics and deep learning has headed to a new era of cardiovascular health management. This innovation has the potential to significantly improve patient health outcomes and transform the way we diagnose and treat heart disease. By using real-time data from mobile ECG systems and leveraging advanced analytics, healthcare professionals can gain unprecedented insights into their patients' cardiovascular health, allows for early detection of abnormalities and personalized treatment planning. In this chapter we have gained insights on signals and waves and various cardiovascular rhythms. We have also run some simulations showing various rhythms .We have shown how an app on smartphone can provide real time data to the user using 5G wifi and Bluetooth and store it in cloud based servers using block diagrams and flowcharts. This data is very easily transferrable to healthcare staff for analysis or during emergency situations. We have shown how deep learning is utilized in the prediction of any untimely heart condition. It consists of learning models and sets. Additionally, we have also calculated the t statistic and the %difference between 2 sets.We have shown how CNN in particular has played a role in classifying ECG signals using a line diagram. We have also shown a number of algorithms to classify heart diseases. Deep learning algorithms can analyze large amounts of ECG data, identifying patterns and abnormalities that might otherwise go unnoticed. Additionally, remote monitoring and remote treatment solutions powered by IoT technology provide convenience for continuous care, improve patient engagement, and reduce the burden on the care system and doctors. In summary, the combination of ECG-based care, IoT, analytics, and deep learning represents a promising future in cardiovascular health that has the potential to save lives, reduce healthcare costs, and promote a healthier and better informed society.

As these technologies continue to advance, we can expect even more innovative solutions to emerge, further revolutionizing the field of cardiovascular care.

References

[1] Kristine Joyce P. Ortiz, John Peter O. Davalos, Elora S. Eusebio and Dominic M. Tucay, IoT: Electrocardiogram (ECG) Monitoring System. 2018.

[2] Gandhi, Bani and Raghava, N.S. Smart ECG Monitoring System Based on IoT. Home Advances in Cognitive Science and Communications Conference Paper. 2023.

[3] Rajkumar, G., Gayathri Devi, T. and Srinivasan, A. Heart disease prediction using IoT based framework and improved deep learning approach: Medical application. 2023.

[4] Devi, A., Matilda, S., Kavya, G., Ananth Kumar, T. and Glorindal, G. IoT-based cardiovascular prediction framework using deep learning algorithms. 2022.

[5] Muhammad Nazrul Islam, Kazi Rafd Raiyan, Shutonu Mitra, M.M. Rushadul Mannan, Tasfa Tasnim et al. Predictis: An IoT and machine learning-based system to predict risk level of cardio-vascular diseases. 2023

[6] Ukil, A., Bandyoapdhyay, S., Puri, C. and Pal, A. IoT healthcare analytics: The importance of anomaly detection. *In:* 2016 IEEE 30th International Conference on Advanced Information Networking and Applications (AINA), pp. 994-997, 2016, March. IEEE.

[7] Banerjee, A., Chakraborty, C., Kumar, A. and Biswas, D. Emerging trends in IoT and big data analytics for biomedical and health care technologies. Handbook of Data Science Approaches for Biomedical Engineering, 121-152, 2020.

[8] Roy, S.S., Roy, A., Samui, P., Gandomi, M. and Gandomi, A.H. Hateful sentiment detection in real-time tweets: An LSTM-based comparative approach. IEEE Transactions on Computational Social Systems. 2023.

[9] Roy, S.S., Pratyush, C. and Barna, C. Predicting ozone layer concentration using multivariate adaptive regression splines, random forest and classification and regression tree. *In:* Soft Computing Applications: Proceedings of the 7th International Workshop Soft Computing Applications (SOFA 2016), Volume 2 7: 140-152, 2018. Springer International Publishing.

[10] Roy, S.S., Gupta, A., Sinha, A. and Ramesh, R. Cancer data investigation using variable precision rough set with flexible classification. *In:* Proceedings of the Second International Conference on Computational Science, Engineering and Information Technology, pp. 472-475, 2012, October.

[11] Bose, A., Roy, S.S., Balas, V.E. and Samui, P. Deep learning for brain computer interfaces. Handbook of Deep Learning Applications, 333-344, 2019.

[12] Roy, S.S. and Taguchi, Y.H. 2021. Identification of genes associated with altered gene expression and m6A profiles during hypoxia using tensor decomposition based unsupervised feature extraction. Scientific Reports, 11(1): 8909.

[13] Chakraborty, C., Bhattacharya, M., Sharma, A.R., Roy, S.S., Islam, M.A., Chakraborty, S. et al. Deep learning research should be encouraged for diagnosis and treatment of antibiotic resistance of microbial infections in treatment associated emergencies in hospitals. International Journal of Surgery, 105: 106857, 2022.

[14] Roy, S.S., Krishna, P.V. and Yenduri, S. Analyzing intrusion detection system: An ensemble based stacking approach. *In:* 2014 IEEE International Symposium on Signal Processing and Information Technology (ISSPIT), 000307-000309, 2014, December. IEEE.

[15] Bandhu, A. and Roy, S.S. Classifying multi-category images using deep learning: A convolutional neural network model. *In:* 2017 2nd IEEE International Conference on Recent Trends in Electronics, Information & Communication Technology (RTEICT), 915-919, 2017, May. IEEE.

[16] Basu, A., Roy, S.S. and Abraham, A. A novel diagnostic approach based on support vector machine with linear kernel for classifying the erythemato-squamous disease. *In:* 2015 International Conference on Computing Communication Control and Automation, 343-347, 2015, February. IEEE.

[17] Pandey, A.K. and Roy, S.S. Natural language generation using sequential models: A survey. Neural Processing Letters, 1-34. 2023.

[18] Mohanty, S., Mohanty, S., Pattnaik, P.K., Vaidya, A. and Hol, A. Smart healthcare analytics using internet of things: An overview. Smart Healthcare Analytics: State of the Art, 1-11, 2022.

[19] An Efficient IoT-Based Patient Monitoring and Heart Disease Prediction System Using Deep Learning Modified Neural Network | IEEE Journals & Magazine | IEEE Xplore. Accessed: Nov. 17, 2023. [Online]. Available: https://ieeexplore.ieee.org/abstract/document/9133567

[20] Ahamed, J., Manan Koli, A., Ahmad, K., Alam Jamal, M. and Gupta, B.B. CDPS-IoT: Cardiovascular disease prediction system based on IoT using machine learning. Jun. 2022, doi: 10.9781/ijimai.2021.09.002

[21] Tuli, S., Nipam Basumatary, Sukhpal Singh Gill, Mohsen Kahani, Rajesh Chand Arya, Gurpreet Singh Wander et al. HealthFog: An ensemble deep learning based Smart Healthcare System for Automatic Diagnosis of Heart Diseases in integrated IoT and fog computing environments. Future Gener. Comput. Syst., 104: 187-200, Mar. 2020, doi: 10.1016/j.future.2019.10.043.

[22] Gheorghe, A., Griffiths, U., Murphy, A., Legido-Quigley, H., Lamptey, P. and Perel, P. The economic burden of cardiovascular disease and hypertension in low- and middle-income countries: A systematic review. BMC Public Health, 18(1): 975, Aug. 2018, doi: 10.1186/s12889-018-5806-x.

CHAPTER
10

Transfer Learning for Multiclass Classification of Bone Marrow Cells

Rishabh Hanselia[1], Dilip Kumar Choubey[1*][0000-0002-1233-7159], Kanchan Bala[2] and Ashutosh Mishra[3]

[1] Department of Computer Science & Engineering, Indian Institute of Information Technology Bhagalpur, Bihar, India

[2] Department of Computer Science & Engineering, Gaya College of Engineering, Gaya, DSTTE, Bihar

[3] Department of Computer Science & Engineering, Thapar Institute of Engineering & Technology, Patiala, Punjab, India

Accurate classification of bone marrow cells for hematological disorder diagnosis faces challenges due to complex morphology and subjectivity in manual assessment. Inconsistencies among experts, time constraints, and intra-observer variability further hinder the process. To address these issues, researchers are working on standardized criteria, improved resources, and AI-based automation. This study rigorously analyzes diverse deep and machine learning techniques in bone marrow cell classification, highlighting their role in modernizing cytology. The authors present their own CNN-based model for digital cytology, achieving a notable 91.66% test accuracy. The study is structured into five main sections: introduction, motivation, related work, material and methods, experimental results, and discussions along with future directions. This research showcases the potential of AI-driven approaches to enhance accuracy and efficiency in bone marrow cell classification, revolutionizing hematological disorder diagnostics.

1. Introduction

Bone marrow cells play a vital role in producing and maturing different types of blood cells. They are made up of platelets (thrombocytes) for clotting, white

*Corresponding author: dkchoubey.cse@iiitbh.ac.in

blood cells (leukocytes) for immunity, and red blood cells (erythrocytes) for oxygen delivery. Hematopoiesis, the process of cell differentiation, occurs within the bone marrow, giving rise to various blood cell types. Analyzing bone marrow cells under a microscope provides valuable diagnostic insights for a wide range of hematological disorders.

Bone marrow cell classification involves categorizing different cell types based on their characteristics and functions. The main types are red blood cells, white blood cells, and platelets. Red blood cells are classified based on developmental stages and hemoglobin content, while white blood cells have subtypes like neutrophils, lymphocytes, monocytes, eosinophils, and basophils. Platelets are categorized by size and granule presence. Accurate classification helps diagnose hematological disorders, done through microscopic examination, immunohistochemistry, and flow cytometry. It aids in assessing cellular composition, identifying abnormal cells, and determining disease stage and severity.

The manual classification of bone marrow cells by humans encounters various obstacles, including subjectivity, variability, complex morphology, time-consuming nature, limited training resources, intra- and inter-observer variability, and error propagation. In response to these challenges, researchers are actively working on the development of automated and AI-based systems. The objective of these methods is to improve bone marrow cell classification efficiency, consistency, and accuracy. By reducing subjectivity, providing standardized results, and addressing the limitations of manual classification, these advancements hold promise for enhancing diagnostic capabilities in the field of hematopathology.

The structure of the manuscript is as distributed: The Motivation is covered in Section 2, the Related Work is covered in Section 3, the Material and Methods are explained in Section 4, the Experimental Results are presented in Section 5, and the Discussion and Future Directions are covered in Section 6.

2. Motivation

Bone marrow cells fulfill a crucial role in the generation and maturation of diverse blood cell types. This encompasses red blood cells, which transport oxygen, white blood cells that engage in immune responses, and platelets essential for blood clotting. Hematopoiesis, occurring within the bone marrow, leads to the emergence of varied blood cell types. The microscopic examination of bone marrow cells yields valuable diagnostic insights for an array of hematological disorders.

The classification of bone marrow cells involves categorizing distinct cell types based on their attributes and functions. Predominant categories include red blood cells, white blood cells, and platelets. Red blood cells are differentiated by developmental stages and hemoglobin content. Meanwhile, white blood cells encompass subtypes such as neutrophils, lymphocytes, monocytes, eosinophils, and basophils. Platelets are categorized by size and granule presence. Precise classification aids in the diagnosis of hematological disorders, contributing to the assessment of cellular composition, identification of abnormal cells, and determination of disease severity.

Manual classification of bone marrow cells faces challenges, including subjectivity, intricate morphology, time intensiveness, limited training resources, and observer variability. Addressing these hurdles, ongoing efforts focus on developing automated AI-based systems. These advancements seek to enhance accuracy, consistency, and efficiency in bone marrow cell classification. By minimizing subjectivity, offering standardized outcomes, and overcoming manual limitations, these innovations hold the potential to advance diagnostic capabilities in the field of hematopathology.

3. Literature Review

Matek et al. (2021) [1] used CNN-based classifiers namely ResNeXt and a sequential network architecture to automate the evaluation of bone marrow cell morphology. Fu et al. (2020) [2] developed Morphogo an automated analysis system based on a 27-layer CNN to classify bone marrow cells. Tayebi et al. (2022) [3] designed end-to-end AI architecture to facilitate AI-enabled computational pathology. Ananthakrishnan et al. (2022) [4] used a Siamese network to perform automated bone marrow cell classification, and also investigated the performance of other machine learning models alongside CNN like CNN + SVM and CNN + XGB Boost. Yu et al. (2023) [5] implemented a DL pipeline namely AMLnet for the purpose of differential diagnosis between AML and bone marrow smears. Based on bone marrow smears, the Image-net pretrained the CNN network and (Wang et al., 2022) [6] automatically distinguished acute myeloid leukemia (AML), myelodysplastic syndrome (MDS), and aplastic anemia (AA) from each other. Choi et al. (2017) [7] used dual-stage CNN with architecture inspired by VGGnet to come up with an automated system for conducting the white blood cell differential count. Song et al. (2018) [8] propose a novel approach in their study, which involves sthe use of a synchronized deep autoencoder network. This network is specifically designed to enable the classification of cells in bone marrow histology images. Chandradevan et al. (2020) [9] generated datasets containing cellular constituents of bone marrow aspirate (BMA) and utilized these datasets to construct a ML algorithm capable of detecting and classifying BMA cells. Kimura et al. (2019) [10] utilized a combination of CNN and XGBoost algorithms to create an automated system with the ability to distinguish myelodysplastic syndrome (MDS) from aplastic anemia (AA). A brand-new DL model named BMSNet was created by Wu et al. (2020) [11] with the intention of helping hematologists read bone marrow smears more quickly and efficiently for disease monitoring.

Liu et al. (2016) [12] employed the R-CNN (Region-based CNN) to create an innovative morphological diagnosis system for the detection of bone marrow cells.

In a similar vein, numerous machine learning algorithms have been employed by researchers to classify diabetes cases. Functional link CNN has been used by Jangir et al. (2021) [26] to classify actual localized diabetic datasets. A non-parametric Friedman statistical test was used for validation. For the classification of diabetes, researchers have used neural networks [27], fuzzy decision trees [28], and kernel function based SVM [29]. Additionally, researchers have used PSO-SVM [28] and GA [27, 29] as feature selection methods, followed by the previously mentioned set of classification approaches, and have obtained good results with feature selection.

Stumpf et al. (2022) [13] used single-cell RNA sequencing data to efficiently map the biology of bone marrow across animals. To identify different cell types in mouse bone marrow, a multiclass logistic regression model was initially developed, and it performed on par with more complex artificial neural networks. Furthermore, the model showed an overall accuracy of 83% in identifying individual human bone marrow cells. To estimate the concentration of ozone gases in the air, three prediction models, Random Forest, Multivariate Adaptive Regression Splines, and CART, were created by Roy et al. (2018) [14]. Following an analysis of the prediction models, it was found that the Multivariate Adaptive Regression Splines model described the dataset more accurately and performed better in terms of accuracy than Random Forest, CART.

The hierarchical framework that was introduced by Wang et al. (2022) [15] consisted of three main components: a deep learning model that quickly localized BM particles and produced ROI for further analysis; a deep learning model based on patches that identified 16 different cell types, including megakaryocytes, mitotic cells, and four stages of erythroblasts that had not been shown in previous studies; and a fast-stitching model that combined patch-based results to produce final outputs. The approach was first evaluated using cross-validation on a dataset including 12,426 annotated cells, yielding a high recall and accuracy of 0.905 ± 0.078 and 0.989 ± 0.006, respectively. It just took 44 seconds to analyze the BM NDC for a whole-slide image (WSI). A second independent dataset including 3005 cells was employed for evaluation in order to gauge the model's generalizability. The results showed that the suggested approach likewise produced excellent recall and accuracy of 0.842 and 0.988, respectively. The various deep-learning algorithms that have been used in BCIs have been explained by Bose et al. (2019) [16], which has improved the devices' performances. Roy et al. (2021) [17] utilized the recently introduced PCA, TD, KTD for unsupervised feature extraction (FE) on a hypoxia dataset. Our results showed that a limited collection of genes associated with altered gene expression and m6A profiles were successfully identified using PCA, TD, and KTD-based unsupervised FE. Furthermore, these techniques showed an enrichment of biological phrases related to hypoxia with increased statistical significance. Roy et al. (2014) [19] utilized the freely available KDD Cup 99 dataset. A highly secure network access is a fundamental requirement in contemporary society. While the majority of IDS automatically collect data, the examination of such data was previously performed manually. It is imperative that an intrusion detection system (IDS) can withstand multiple intrusions without compromising its performance—this capability is referred to as multiple attack stability. If, after detecting an intrusion, the system becomes sluggish or experiences breakdowns, the IDS loses its value to the organization. Additionally, if attackers are aware of the IDS's poor performance, they could potentially gain control over the entire network. Roy et al. (2023) [20] suggested a method for identifying hate speech. This work proposed a TF-IDF vectorized hate speech detection model based on LSTM. Comparisons were performed using the following models: artificial neural network (ANN), logistic regression from transformers (BERT), SVM, NB, LR, XGBoost, RF, and k -NN. Using the Twitter API, a real-time data stream of a popular subject was gathered and divided into 02 classes: hate speech and non-hate speech, in order to validate and authenticate the proposed work. The LSTM achieved F 1 score, precision, and recall of 0.98, 0.99, and 0.98, respectively. It was shown that LSTM outperformed other models in terms of accuracy when it came to identifying hateful sentiments, with an accuracy rate of 97%. The study of leukemia that was previously provided by Parthvi et al. (2020) [21] used manual microscopic evaluation of the sample slides. However, manual diagnostic methods required a lot of time, were less precise, and were prone to mistakes brought on by a variety of human variables, including stress and exhaustion. It was decided that clustering and classification techniques were required in order to help physicians uncover possible flaws and inaccuracies. As a result, the writers thoroughly examined and analyzed a large number of research publications, with a primary focus on leukemia classification algorithms. This review article's primary objective was to examine and contrast various approaches used in the treatment of leukemia. Choubey et al. (2023) [22] presented a fully automated CNN-based model for the identification of malaria in blood smear micrographs. The algorithm proposed in our study demonstrated a ninety-six percent accuracy rate in detecting malarial parasites from microscopic images. This accuracy can be further enhanced with training and testing on larger datasets. The conventional method for diagnosing malaria involves a competent technician visually analyzing a blood smear under a microscope to identify parasitized red blood cells. The diagnosis relies on the experience and knowledge of the individual conducting the inspection, making it time-consuming and, in rare instances, susceptible to human errors. The research was conducted in two stages: Stage one focused on dataset summarization, while Stage two addressed the implementation and evaluation of the proposed algorithm. Agarwal et al. (2023) [23] have designed a medical dispensary box by using an improved version of IoT. It is more useful for senior people and those who are having issues in remembering medicine quantities and times.

Choubey et al. (2020) [24] proposed an application to real time crops which improves production. Choubey et al. (2022) [25] proposed an IoT based machine learning algorithm for precision cultivation of crops. The dataset was obtained from Bassi village, Jaipur, Rajasthan, India.

A summary of the previous research paper is shown in Table 1.

Table 1. Summary of the existing works for Bone Marrow Cells

Paper Reference no.	Dataset Used	Methods Used	Advantages	Future Scope/ Limitations	Performance	Purpose
[1]	A collection of single-cell images, meticulously annotated by experts, was amassed. These images were derived from 961 patients who received diagnoses for different hematological diseases at the MLL Munich Leukemia Laboratory during the period from 2011 to 2013	CNN-based classifiers: ResNeXt, sequential network architecture	The proposed model outperforms feature-based classifiers	To decrease the significance of label noise in the evaluation, techniques like semi-supervised or unsupervised methods can be employed. These methods have previously demonstrated their efficacy in processes such as erythrocyte assessment and cell cycle reconstruction.	0.95 precision (tolerant), 0.92 precision (strict), 0.85 recall (tolerant) and 0.71 recall (strict) were the highest among all the classes	To make progress in automating the evaluation of bone marrow (BM) cell morphology using cutting-edge image classification algorithms
[2]	A total of 230 cases of bone marrow direct aspirate smears were obtained from the historical archives and daily examinations at Xinqiao Hospital of the Army Medical University. The dataset	Automated analysis system (Morphogo) utilizing a 27-layer CNN	The utilization of digital image acquisition and automated cell image analysis facilitates the identification and display of immature cells, dysplastic cells, model exhibited	To enhance the capabilities of the AI system, it is crucial to provide more extensive training on a large-scale dataset that encompasses diverse and representative cell types, The current instrument faces limitations in	Accuracy 85.7%, sensitivity 69.4, and specificity 97.2%	To investigate its possible clinical implications, a novel AI system was developed to automatically classify bone marrow cells.

(*Contd.*)

Table 1. (*Contd.*)

Paper Reference no.	Dataset Used	Methods Used	Advantages	Future Scope/ Limitations	Performance	Purpose
	comprised 76 male and 154 female patients. The data collection period spanned from November 26, 2018, to January 30, 2019		and blasts in bone marrow smears. Moreover, this instrument offers a novel workflow and practicality that can benefit any hematology laboratory. By introducing a digital workflow, the efficiency of bone marrow smears can be enhanced, while ensuring a standardized examination process.	capturing comprehensive morphological details of erythroblasts due to its inability to focus accurately on small-sized erythroblasts, For diagnostic purposes, the identification and differentiation of blasts in morphological analysis present another significant challenge that requires attention		
[3]	Digital whole slide images (WSI) were obtained and processed in a de-identified manner. The images were annotated solely with a diagnosis, covering a one-	Automated end-to-end AI architecture consisting of A DenseNet model is employed to select ROI (Region of	An innovative end-to-end AI architecture was introduced, specifically designed for automated bone marrow cytology. This exceptional	The models suffer from overfitting of the local dataset. The availability of annotated publicly accessible or academic digital pathology datasets, especially in	Accuracy 0.97, ROC (AUC) 0.99, Precision 0.75, F1-Score 0.78 average, 0.31 Log-average miss rate	The aim is to facilitate AI-enabled computational pathology, which, in turn, can assist clinicians

	year timeframe and involving a total of 1247 patients	Interest) tiles, while a YOLO model is utilized for detecting and assigning class probabilities	demonstration, demonstrating excellent precision and accuracy in object categorization and ROI detection in a range of clinical validation scenarios. It has the potential to contribute to improved efficiency and accuracy in hematology diagnosis, thereby supporting the integration of AI-enabled computational pathology.	the field of hematopathology workflows and aspirate cytology, is still limited. As a result, external validation was not possible due to the scarcity of such resources.		in making diagnoses that are both more efficient and accurate.
[4]	A collection of 170,000 cell images, annotated by experts, was compiled from bone marrow smears of 945 patients diagnosed with various hematological disorders	Siamese network, CNN + SVM and CNN + XGB Boost	Instead of relying solely on feature extraction from individual images, the approach emphasizes the assessment of	In future implementation, the use of YOLO and Grad-CAM methods will be employed to target the ROI within a single cell image, aiming to	Accuracy 32% (CNN + SVM), Accuracy 28% (CNN + XGB), Accuracy 91%, Validation Accuracy 84%, Weighted	The objective is to discover a method to eliminate the influence of class imbalance in training a deep neural

(*Contd.*)

Table 1. (*Contd.*)

Paper Reference no.	Dataset Used	Methods Used	Advantages	Future Scope/ Limitations	Performance	Purpose
s			similarity and dissimilarity between images of the same and different class labels.	deduce the reliance on convolutional units for encoding generation. Furthermore, diverse image augmentation algorithms will be explored to address the potential impact of class imbalance on accuracy	average Recall 92%, and Weighted Average Recall for validation 91% (Siamese neural)	network, ultimately achieving a significantly high level of overall accuracy.
[5]	An extensive database was established via a retrospective dual-center investigation carried out between 2010 and 2021, containing 8245 bone marrow smear images from 651 participants.	AMLnet, a deep-learning pipeline	On the test dataset, the AI system outperformed junior human experts and produced results that were on par with senior experts at the patient level. This suggests that cytomorphological pathologists could use it as a quick prescreening and decision support tool.	The performance of AMLnet will be assessed in extensive and diverse cohorts of hematological malignancy patients from various regions	AUC 0.885 (image level) and 0.921 (patient level)	The objective was to develop a deep-learning pipeline using bone marrow smear images. The pipeline was designed to not only distinguish between individuals with acute myeloid leukemia

						(AML) and healthy people, as well as correctly distinguishing various AML subtypes.
[6]	American Society of Hematology (ASH) Image Bank: In total, 115 bone marrow smears from the ASH Image Bank and 432 bone marrow smears from the clinic were used in this investigation.	Image-net pretrained model of CNN showcasing 2 output layers: two classifications and three classifications	No previous reports have addressed this specific classification task. The robust performance of the model on the external validation set provides evidence that it remains effective and reliable, despite the limitations and constraints	In future research, it is crucial to not only concentrate on disease identification but also on exploring disease progression. The study's sample size was relatively small, highlighting the necessity for larger-scale investigations in the future. Disparities continued between the augmented samples and the individual samples even after data augmentation techniques were used to improve the samples, which might have an impact on our study's findings. The study	AUC 0.985, Accuracy 91.4%, Sensitivity 0.992 (two classification), AUC 0.968, Accuracy 92.9%, Sensitivity 0.857 (three classifications)	To design a convolutional neural network (CNN) model capable of automatically distinguishing between aplastic anemia (AA), myelodysplastic syndrome (MDS), and acute myeloid leukemia (AML) based on bone marrow smears

(*Contd.*)

Table 1. *(Contd.)*

Paper Reference no.	Dataset Used	Methods Used	Advantages	Future Scope/ Limitations	Performance	Purpose
				was unable to assess the different subtypes of acute myeloid leukemia (AML) and myelodysplastic syndrome (MDS) due to the restricted sample number available in the ASH Image Bank. There were issues with the study's ability to pinpoint the characteristics of cases that the model misclassified or that were inconsistent. This resulted from a lack of understanding of the particular properties that deep learning was able to extract from a single image. Due to the lack of pertinent patient information		

				in the database, it was not possible to analyze the differences between patients in the hospital and those in the database. This limitation could impact the generalizability of our findings and the extrapolation of results to a broader patient population		
[7]	The collection of 2,174 patch images for training and testing purposes was carried out at the Department of Laboratory Medicine, Seoul National University Hospital	Dual-stage CNN with architecture inspired by VGGnet containing 16 layers.	The suggested approach demonstrated remarkable classification efficacy, proficiently classifying unprocessed images without requiring manual feature extraction or single cell segmentation. Rotation and location invariance were proved by the method using Convolutional	The model's classification capabilities should include a complete list of white blood cell (WBC) types, such as plasma cells and lymphocytes, along with specific disease models like different stages of leukemia. This comprehensive approach ensures accurate and effective classification, enabling improved analysis and diagnosis in the field of hematology. The network used in	Accuracy 97.06%, Precision 97.13%, Recall 97.06%, and F-1 score 97.1%	To develop an automated system for conducting the white blood cell differential count, effectively minimizing variations in results obtained by different hematologists

(*Contd.*)

Table 1. *(Contd.)*

Paper Reference no.	Dataset Used	Methods Used	Advantages	Future Scope/ Limitations	Performance	Purpose
			Neural Networks (CNN). These results highlight the suggested method's potential as an automated white blood cell differential count system, presenting encouraging progress in the area.	this study was originally designed for general image classification tasks. However, a specific architecture is necessary to cater to the unique requirements of the study.		
[8]	A collection of 52 H&E-stained histopathological bone marrow trephine biopsy images was obtained from 5 essential thrombocythemia (ET) and 5 profibrotic primary myelofibrosis (PMF) patient cases. The images were sourced from University Hospitals Coventry and Warwickshire (UHCW)	Synchronized deep autoencoder network, curve-support Gaussian model, neighborhood selection mechanism	Presents a unique approach by introducing a novel neighborhood selection mechanism that significantly enhances the detection and classification accuracy . The model employs comparable high-level feature representations, enabling a reduction in the network's layer complexity	In the future, there is a scope to enhance the proposed network by extending its capabilities to perform additional tasks like segmentation and classification. This can be achieved by incorporating convolutional layers, which will contribute to improved performance and reduced training time.	Precision 0.9266, Recall 0.9674, and F-1 score 0.9466 (against other methods). Precision 0.8712, Recall 0.8879, and F-1 score 0.8795 against other DL frameworks)	To address the inevitable rise in computational complexity during the training steps in digital histology, the objective is to develop a model that effectively reduces this burden

[9]	Wright-stained bone marrow aspirate (BMA) smear samples from 17 patients were obtained for standard patient treatment. These smears were scanned for additional analysis after being deidentified. From June to August of 2015, the smears were consistently prepared by the bone marrow laboratory at Emory University Hospital.	Faster Region-Based Convolutional Network	The findings of this study have the potential to greatly aid in the diagnosis and prognosis of various diseases, thereby making a significant impact on clinical practice	The classification accuracies reported for disease cases in this study may benefit from improvement since the training did not include cells from these cases. The utilization of small regions of interest (ROIs) in this study was biased towards selecting areas with improved cytologic preservation. Investigating the potential advantages of utilizing higher resolution scanned images will be valuable, especially as the feasibility of acquiring and storing these large digitized images increases in the clinical setting. The study has not yet defined specific performance criteria for the clinical validation of this emerging method, which is still in its early stages of development	AUC 0.959 (detection), AUC 0.982 (classification)	To develop an automated system for performing differential cell counts (DCCs) on Bone Marrow Aspirate (BMA) samples which play a crucial role in accurately classifying hematologic disorders

(Contd.)

Table 1. *(Contd.)*

Paper Reference no.	Dataset Used	Methods Used	Advantages	Future Scope/ Limitations	Performance	Purpose
[10]	A dataset of 3,261 peripheral blood (PB) smears was created at Junten-do University Hospital in Tokyo, Japan, between 2017 and 2018. Off them, 1,165 were from patients with different hematological illnesses.	The system utilized a DLS for image recognition based on convolutional neural networks (CNNs) and employed an EGB algorithm for decision-making, known as XGBoost.	The authors successfully developed the first CNN-based automated initial diagnostic system for myelodysplastic syndromes (MDS) using peripheral blood (PB) smears. This groundbreaking system has the potential to be adapted and utilized for the development of automated diagnostic systems for a wide range of hematological disorders.	While achieving an accuracy of over 90% in automated MDS diagnosis, it is important to note that our system is still considered adjunctive in its nature. Only a small number of samples and one center were used in this investigation. Because of this, its possible that the training sample patterns employed might not accurately reflect all possible population variations. There was only one DLS, CNN, and XGBoost combination used in the study; no other possible combinations or variants were investigated.	Sensitivity 93.5% specificity 96.0% (DLS), sensitivity 96.2% specificity 100%, AUC 0.990 (MDS)	The objective of this study was to develop deep convolutional neural networks that can aid in distinguishing between myelodysplastic syndrome (MDS) and aplastic anemia (AA).

[11]	During the period from January 1, 2016, to December 31, 2018, a total of 122 bone marrow smears were captured through photography.	BMSNet, a convolutional neural network with the YOLO v3 architecture	BMSNet exhibited a performance similar to that of the hematologists.	The performance of BMSNet was compared in the study to that of just six visiting staff members. The captured photos in the study were taken by experienced technicians. However, using an automatic slide scanner is recommended for an optimal process to eliminate the operator effect.	AUC 0.948 (5% of blasts), AUC 0.942 (20% of blasts)	To create a deep learning model called BMSNet, aimed at assisting hematologists in interpreting bone marrow smears for expedited diagnosis and disease monitoring.
[12]	The dataset used in the study consisted of a total of 4,451 authentic images of bone marrow cells.	Faster Region-Convolutional Neural Network (R-CNN)	The newly developed diagnostic system demonstrated a faster response speed compared to that of trained diagnostic experts.	The model was trained using a dataset consisting of 4,451 fields from a limited number of 70 patients. Since the cell types included in the dataset are sourced from a single center, there is a possibility of bias towards the specific population and imaging machines used in that center. The model may face challenges in effectively learning from rare samples.	Recall 0.710, precision 0.496, F1-score 0.575	The objective of the study was to develop a novel morphological diagnosis system for the detection of bone marrow cells using a deep learning object detection framework.

As shown in Table 1, Figs. 1 to 7 show graphical performance representations of the models under study. Figure 1 represents accuracy; Figures 2 and 3 represent AUC, Precision, and Recall; Figures 5 and 6 represent F1 Score, Sensitivity, and Specificity, respectively. Figure 1 present the performance in terms of Accuracy for the mentioned models.

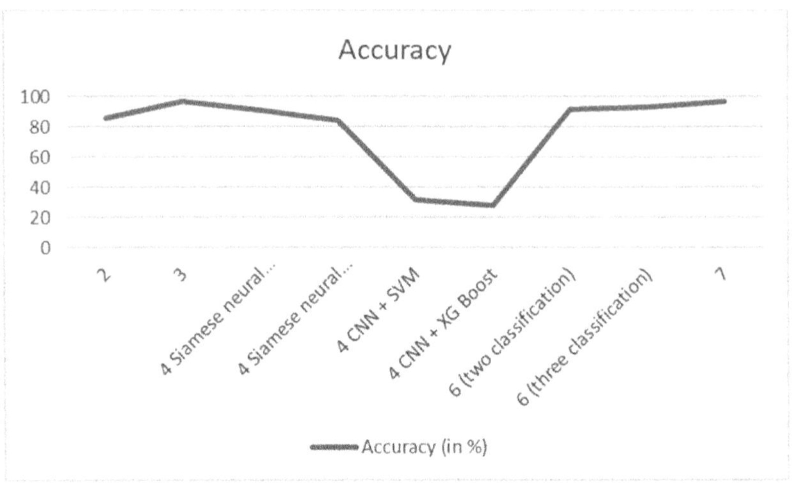

Figure 1. Accuracy for the models

Figure 2 present the performance in terms of AUC for the mentioned models.

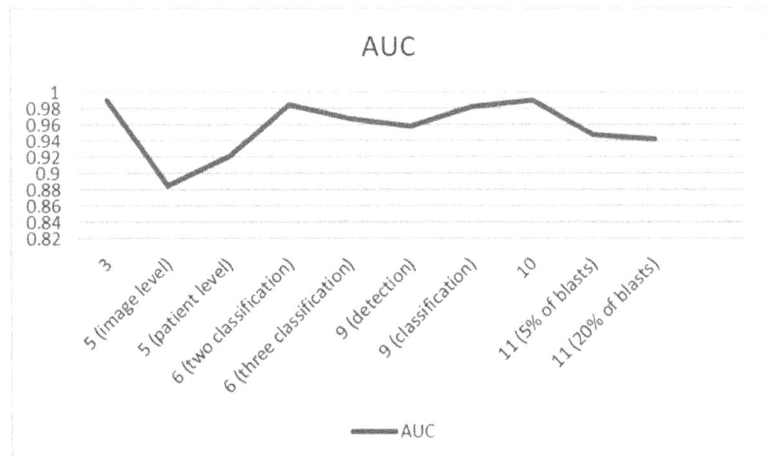

Figure 2. AUC for the models

Figure 3 present the performance in terms of Precision for the mentioned models.

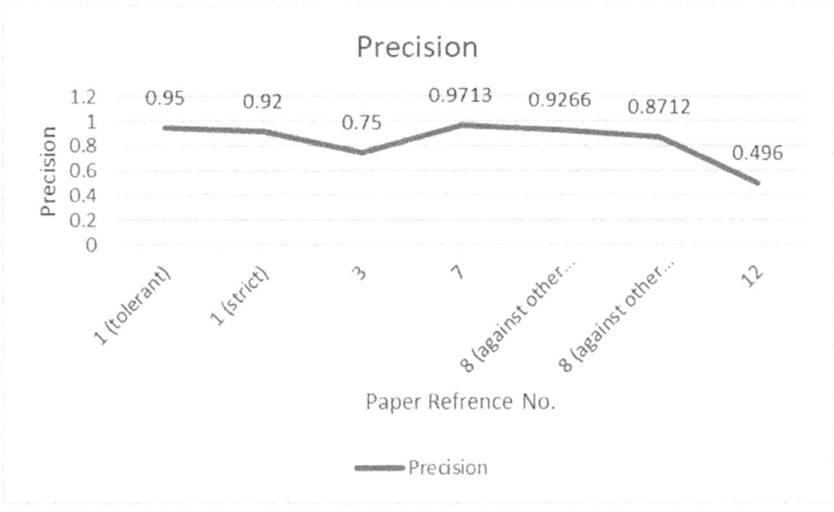

Figure 3. Precision for the models

Figure 4 present the performance in terms of Recall for the mentioned models.

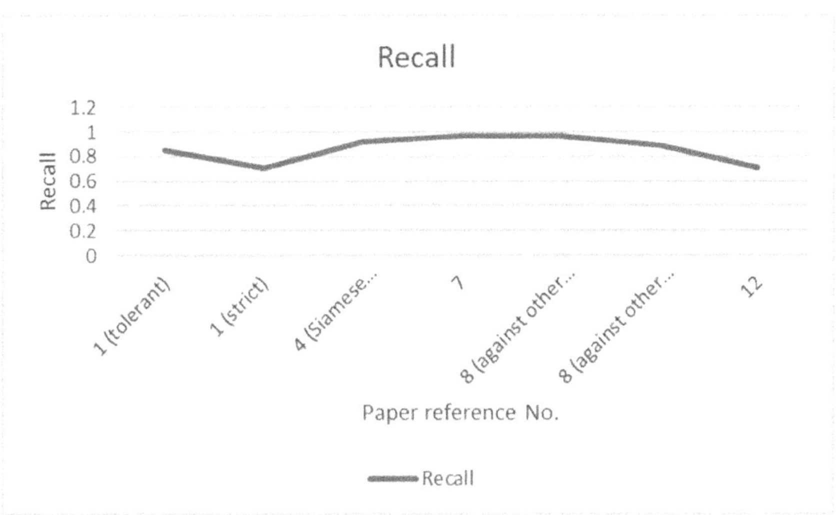

Figure 4. Recall for the models

Figure 5 present the performance in terms of F1 Score for the mentioned models. Figure 6 present the performance in terms of Sensitivity for the mentioned models.

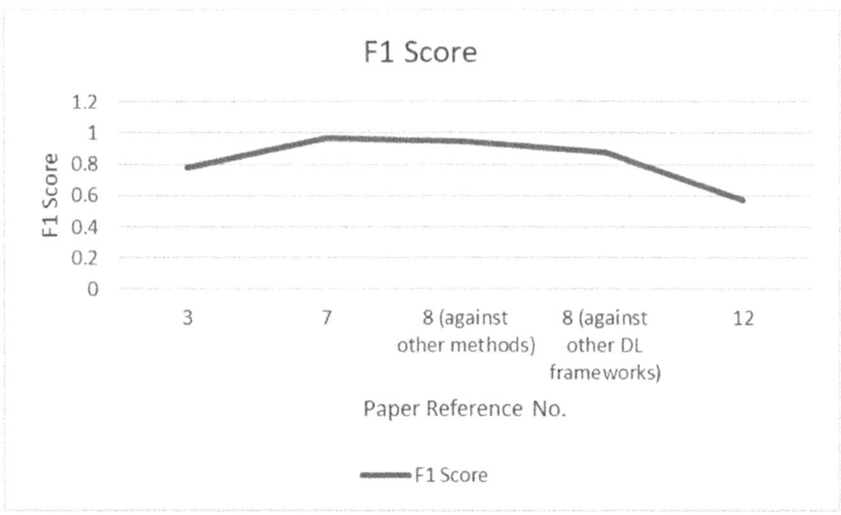

Figure 5. F1 Score for the models

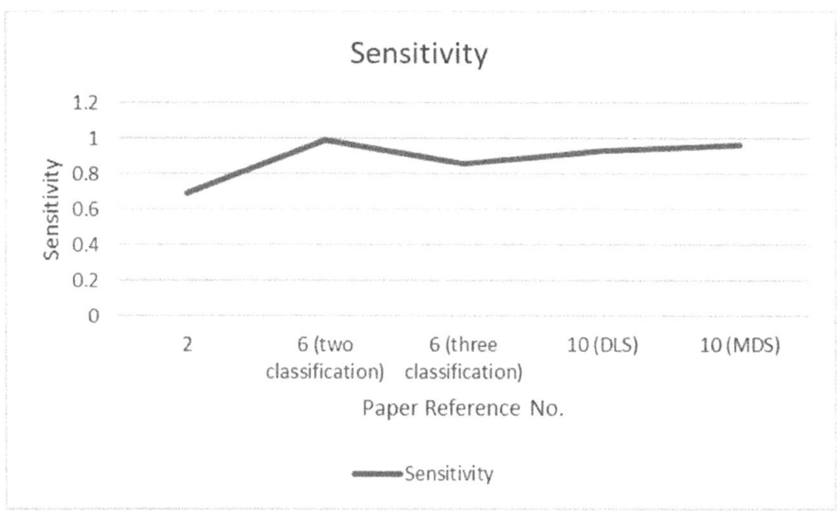

Figure 6. Sensitivity for the models

Figure 7 present the performance in terms of Specificity for the mentioned models.

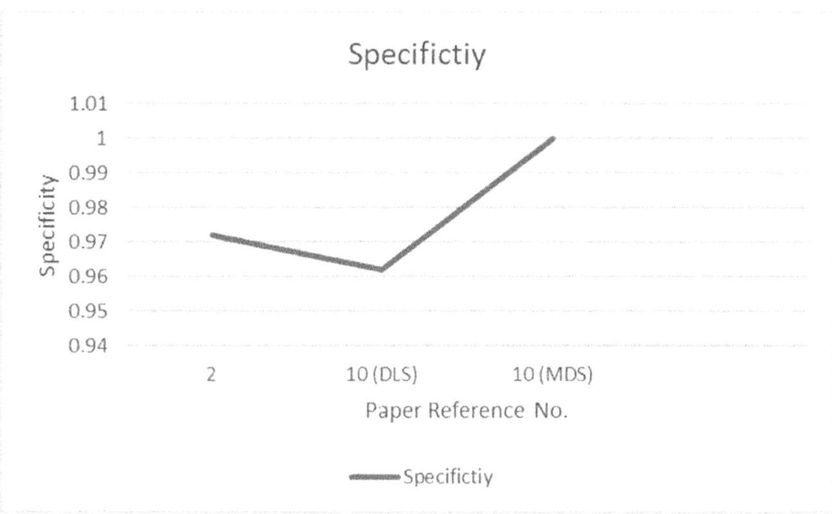

Figure 7. Specificity for the models

4. Material and Methods

This section demonstrates the assortment of tools and resources employed in the construction of the multiclass classification model for bone marrow cells.

4.1 Tools Used

The various tools used are stated below:

- **Python:** Python, a high-level programming language established in 1991, emphasizes readability and versatility. Its rich standard library and third-party frameworks like NumPy, TensorFlow, and Django empower tasks spanning data analysis, machine learning, and web development. Python's popularity thrives due to its simplicity, broad community, and cross-platform compatibility.
- **Jupyter Notebook:** This is, an open-source web app, facilitates live code, visualizations, and text sharing. Supporting 40+ languages, it enables interactive coding, data exploration, and collaboration. Its browser-based interface ensures access from anywhere, while multimedia integration enhances presentation. With a dashboard for organization, Jupyter Notebook empowers reproducible, interactive computational notebooks.
- **Numpy:** NumPy, a core Python library, empowers large array handling and mathematical functions. Vital in data science, machine learning, and more, it efficiently performs numerical operations and seamlessly integrates with Pandas, Matplotlib, and SciPy. NumPy notebooks offer interactive data exploration and analysis, making it indispensable for research and computation.

- **Pandas:** Pandas, an open-source Python library, excels in data manipulation and analysis. Featuring DataFrames for structured data and Series for one-dimensional arrays, it seamlessly handles missing data and integrates with NumPy, Matplotlib, and scikit-learn. Pandas is a pivotal tool for diverse fields, offering efficient data handling, exploration, and modeling.
- **Sklearn:** Scikit-learn (sklearn) is a prominent open-source machine learning library for Python. With diverse algorithms, it handles classification, regression, clustering, and more. Leveraging NumPy, SciPy, and Matplotlib, it offers efficiency, consistency, and ease. Scikit-learn simplifies model implementation, providing tools for preprocessing, evaluation, and visualization, making it a top choice in machine learning.
- **Matplotlib:** Matplotlib, a popular data visualization library for Python, offers versatile tools for creating static, interactive, and animated visualizations. It supports various plot types, customizations, and seamless integration with NumPy and Pandas. With high-level and object-oriented interfaces, Matplotlib empowers both simple and complex visualizations, engaging a broad community for learning and solutions.
- **Tensorflow:** TensorFlow, developed by Google, is a popular open-source framework for deep learning model building and training. It employs computational graphs for efficient parallel processing and supports diverse neural network architectures. TensorFlow offers high-level simplicity through Keras and advanced customization with low-level APIs. Its strong community support and distributed computing capability contribute to its prominence in AI and deep learning.

4.2 Workflow

The work flow is as follows:

1. Importing of necessary libraries
2. Loading of dataset – Image folder
3. Augmentation of data
4. Setting up the various parameters of the model
5. Checking the batch for test
6. Building of Model
7. Display of the model summary – checking purpose
8. Training of the model
9. Presentation of the performance of the model

In this study, a multiclass classification task was conducted using transfer learning on a dataset consisting of images of bone marrow cells belonging to different cell types. The data was prepared and preprocessed to ensure its compatibility with a convolutional neural network (CNN) model, specifically EfficientNetB5.

EfficientNetB5, a pre-trained CNN model called for its effectiveness in image classification tasks, was employed to leverage its learned features and optimize the classification performance on the bone marrow cell dataset.

All experiments were conducted within the Jupyter Notebook environment, utilizing Python 3.9 as the programming language. Jupyter Notebook provides an interactive and collaborative platform for executing code, analyzing results, and documenting the experimental process.

By performing multiclass classification using transfer learning, this work aimed to accurately classify bone marrow cell images into their respective cell types. Transfer learning allows the model to leverage knowledge learned from a large and diverse dataset, enhancing its ability to generalize and make accurate predictions on the bone marrow cell dataset.

Python 3.9 was chosen as the programming language due to its extensive support for deep learning libraries and image processing capabilities. The combination of Jupyter Notebook and Python 3.9 provided an efficient and effective environment for conducting the experiments, analyzing the results, and documenting the findings.

In summary, this study employed transfer learning using the EfficientNetB5 model to perform multiclass classification on a dataset of bone marrow cell images. The choice of Jupyter Notebook and Python 3.9 as the implementation tools facilitated the experimental process and enabled accurate classification of bone marrow cell types.

4.3 Dataset

The dataset used in this study comprises more than 170,000 de-identified bone marrow cells obtained from the smears of 945 patients. These cells were stained using the May-Grünwald-Giemsa/Pappenheim staining technique. The cohort represented a diverse range of hematological diseases, reflecting the samples collected by a specialized laboratory focused on leukemia diagnostics.

The image acquisition process involved using a 40x magnification capable brightfield microscope and oil immersion. All samples were processed at the Munich Leukemia Laboratory (MLL). The scanning of the samples was performed using equipment developed by Fraunhofer IIS. Subsequently, the captured images underwent post-processing using software developed at Helmholtz Munich.

The dataset used is anonymized, ensuring the privacy and confidentiality of the patients' information. The expert annotation of the cells provides valuable insights and annotations for analysis and research purposes.

The utilization of this comprehensive dataset enables researchers to explore and analyze various aspects related to hematological diseases, leveraging the expertise and advancements in imaging technology from renowned institutions and laboratories.

4.4 Algorithm Description

The cutting-edge convolutional neural network (CNN) architecture known as EfficientNetB5 has drawn a lot of interest and demonstrated outstanding performance in a variety of computer vision applications, such as semantic segmentation, object identification, and picture classification. It is part of the EfficientNet family of models, which are designed to provide high accuracy with a great reduction in parameters when compared to conventional models.

EfficientNetB5 was introduced by Mingxing Tan and Quoc V. Le in their 2019 paper titled "EfficientNet: Rethinking Model Scaling for Convolutional Neural Networks". The main idea behind EfficientNetB5 is to scale up the baseline architecture by applying compound scaling to depth, width, and resolution dimensions. This scaling strategy ensures that the model's performance is improved while maintaining efficiency in terms of computational resources and memory requirements.

The "B5" in EfficientNetB5 refers to the scaling coefficient used for the architecture. EfficientNet models are generally denoted by a compound scaling coefficient, where higher values indicate larger and more powerful models. EfficientNetB5 has a higher coefficient compared to its predecessors, such as EfficientNetB0 or EfficientNetB3.

EfficientNetB5 achieves its efficiency and performance through a combination of architectural advancements and scaling techniques. The architecture of EfficientNetB5 follows a similar pattern as other CNNs, consisting of multiple stacked convolutional layers with non-linear activations, followed by pooling layers and fully connected layers for classification. However, it incorporates several notable features:

1. **Depthwise Separable Convolution:** Depthwise separable convolutions, used by EfficientNetB5, divide the conventional convolutional operation into two stages: a depthwise convolution that applies a single filter to each input channel, and a pointwise convolution that merges the result of the depthwise convolution across channels. This strategy reduces the number of model parameters as well as the computational complexity.
2. **Inverted Residuals with Linear Bottlenecks:** Inspired by the MobileNetV2 architecture, EfficientNetB5 uses inverted residuals, where a bottleneck layer with a reduced number of channels is followed by a linear projection layer, increasing the model's representational power while keeping the computational cost low.
3. **Efficient Scaling Coefficient:** EfficientNetB5 incorporates a scaling coefficient that determines the depth, width, and resolution of the model. The scaling coefficients are derived using a compound scaling method that maintains a balance between these dimensions. This approach allows the model to achieve higher accuracy without significantly increasing the computational requirements.

4. **Efficient Compound Scaling:** EfficientNetB5 leverages compound scaling to optimize the model's performance. Instead of scaling each dimension independently, compound scaling considers the trade-offs among different dimensions, enabling more efficient use of resources. It ensures that the model's depth, width, and resolution are scaled proportionally, resulting in improved accuracy.

The EfficientNetB5 model has been trained on large-scale datasets, such as ImageNet, and has demonstrated excellent performance in various image classification challenges. Its efficiency and high accuracy make it a popular choice for computer vision applications, particularly when computational resources are limited. Researchers and practitioners often adopt EfficientNetB5 as a strong baseline model for transfer learning or as a starting point for further customization and fine-tuning to suit specific tasks and datasets.

5. Experimental Results

This section shows the experimental results and analysis for the various experiments discussed in materials and methods and also explains the performance metrics for the same after implementing algorithms and models.

5.1 Diagnostic Performance Description

- **Training and Testing Loss Graph:** This graph illustrates how a model's error changes during training and testing. Training involves minimizing the loss function, reflecting the gap between predictions and targets. Decreasing training loss signifies learning progress. Testing loss, evaluated on separate data, gauges generalization. Rising testing loss while training loss falls suggests overfitting. This visual aid aids model assessment, highlights overfitting, and guides optimization decisions for enhanced accuracy and generalization.
- **Training and Testing Accuracy Graph:** This graph illustrates a model's performance evolution during training and testing. Training involves minimizing loss while computing accuracy on training data. The graph tracks increasing training accuracy as the model learns to classify training instances better. Subsequently, testing accuracy is evaluated on unseen data, revealing the model's generalization. Initial testing accuracy growth is expected, but decline or plateau while training accuracy rises indicates overfitting. This visualization guides optimization decisions and reveals the model's learning and generalization prowess.

5.2 Results

The experimental results for the survivability prediction of a patient undergoing bone marrow transplant are shown in this section.

Table 2 represents the model performance during the training period, the change in performance of the model over the epochs have been represented.

Table 2. Model Performance History

Epoch	Loss	Accuracy	v_loss	v_acc	LR	Next LR	Monitor	% Improv	Duration
1/40	9.184	57.155	11.55479	48.485	0.001	0.001	Accuracy	0	849.28
2/40	7.678	86.542	9.72927	57.576	0.001	0.001	Accuracy	51.42	647.26
3/40	6.819	93.101	8.00508	61.364	0.001	0.001	val_loss	17.72	649.89
4/40	6.209	95.145	6.98767	69.697	0.001	0.001	val_loss	12.71	627.93
5/40	5.656	97.189	6.0784	76.515	0.001	0.001	val_loss	13.01	606.34
6/40	5.15	98.637	5.37474	84.091	0.001	0.001	val_loss	11.58	591.1
7/40	4.713	98.211	4.8567	85.606	0.001	0.001	val_loss	9.64	566.23
8/40	4.298	98.893	4.4501	87.879	0.001	0.001	val_loss	8.37	564.04
9/40	3.923	98.893	4.04264	86.364	0.001	0.001	val_loss	9.16	585.79
10/40	3.58	99.063	3.70436	89.394	0.001	0.001	val_loss	8.37	1041.73
11/40	3.269	99.148	3.39633	88.636	0.001	0.001	val_loss	832	523.13
12/40	2.981	99.574	3.12081	89.394	0.001	0.001	val_loss	8.11	530.3
13/40	2.719	99.744	2.85188	89.394	0.001	0.001	val_loss	8.62	536.59
14/40	2.489	99.574	2.61199	90.909	0.001	0.001	val_loss	8.41	507.99

15/40	2.274	99.915	2.43904	89.394	0.001	0.001	val_loss	6.62	522.57
16/40	2.084	99.574	2.2402	89.394	0.001	0.001	val_loss	8.15	508.2
17/40	1.908	99.574	2.07439	90.152	0.001	0.001	val_loss	7.4	515.48
18/40	1.744	99.574	1.89762	90.152	0.001	0.001	val_loss	8.52	522.44
19/40	1.595	99.744	1.78942	89.394	0.001	0.001	val_loss	5.7	519.28
20/40	1.452	100	1.64133	89.394	0.001	0.001	val_loss	8.28	513.66
21/40	1.343	99.744	1.54562	89.394	0.001	0.001	val_loss	5.83	519.36
22/40	1.235	99.915	1.44333	88.636	0.001	0.001	val_loss	6.62	512.63
23/40	1.121	100	1.31968	90.152	0.001	0.001	val_loss	8.57	512.6
24/40	1.034	99.744	1.2142	90.909	0.001	0.001	val_loss	7.99	510.2
25/40	0.966	99.744	1.15664	90.152	0.001	0.001	val_loss	4.74	513.62
26/40	0.879	99.83	1.07645	90.152	0.001	0.001	val_loss	6.93	512.9
27/40	0.811	100	1.044	90.152	0.001	0.001	val_loss	3.01	512.49
28/40	0.746	100	0.97865	89.394	0.001	0.001	val_loss	6.26	514.33
29/40	0.691	99.915	0.91845	90.909	0.001	0.001	val_loss	6.15	511.34
30/40	0.648	99.915	0.87526	90.909	0.001	0.001	val_loss	4.7	508.86

(Contd.)

Table 2. *(Contd.)*

Epoch	Loss	Accuracy	v_loss	v_acc	LR	Next LR	Monitor	% Improv	Duration
31/40	0.595	99.915	0.83522	89.394	0.001	0.001	val_loss	4.57	510.92
32/40	0.555	99.83	0.76996	90.909	0.001	0.001	val_loss	7.81	510.51
33/40	0.519	99.915	0.73045	91.667	0.001	0.001	val_loss	5.13	516.51
34/40	0.484	99.83	0.71953	89.394	0.001	0.001	val_loss	1.5	517.46
35/40	0.452	99.915	0.70442	88.636	0.001	0.001	val_loss	2.1	509.86
36/40	0.422	100	0.64993	89.394	0.001	0.001	val_loss	7.74	527.84
37/40	0.396	99.915	0.63923	89.394	0.001	0.001	val_loss	1.65	515.86
38/40	0.375	100	0.59471	91.667	0.001	0.001	val_loss	6.97	512.49
39/40	0.349	100	0.57408	91.667	0.001	0.001	val_loss	3.47	510.43
40/40	0.333	99.915	0.56167	91.667	0.001	0.001	val_loss	2.16	510.04

Table 3 represents the model performance scores. Training and Testing scores have been presented in the table.

Table 3. Train and test scores

Train Loss	0.2929128110408783
Train Accuracy	1.0
Test Loss	0.5616690516471863
Test Accuracy	0.9166666865348816

Figures 8 and 9 represent the model's performance during the training period and the change in performance of the algorithm over the epochs in graphical form respectively. Figure 8 shows the performance loss during training and testing over the epochs.

Figure 9 shows the model accuracy for training and testing over the epochs.

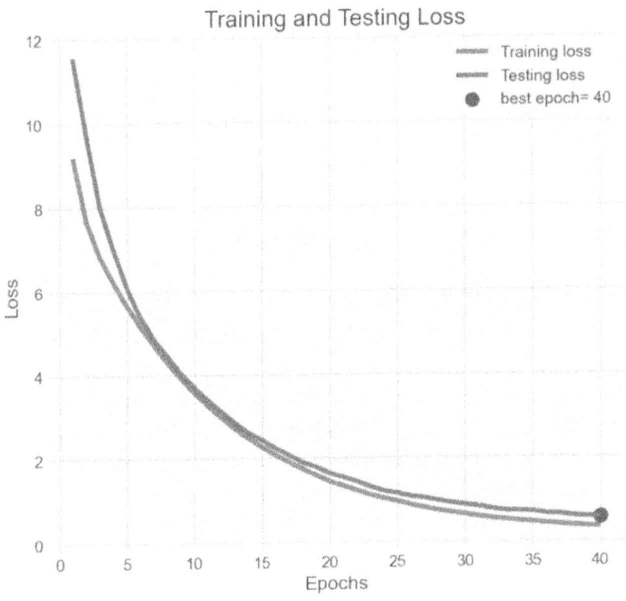

Figure 8. Loss graph of training and testing

6. Discussions and Future Directions

The dataset comprised over 170,000 bone marrow cell images, categorized into directories by labels. After organizing and resizing to 224 × 224 pixels, a 90% training and 10% testing split was applied with a batch size of 40. Utilizing

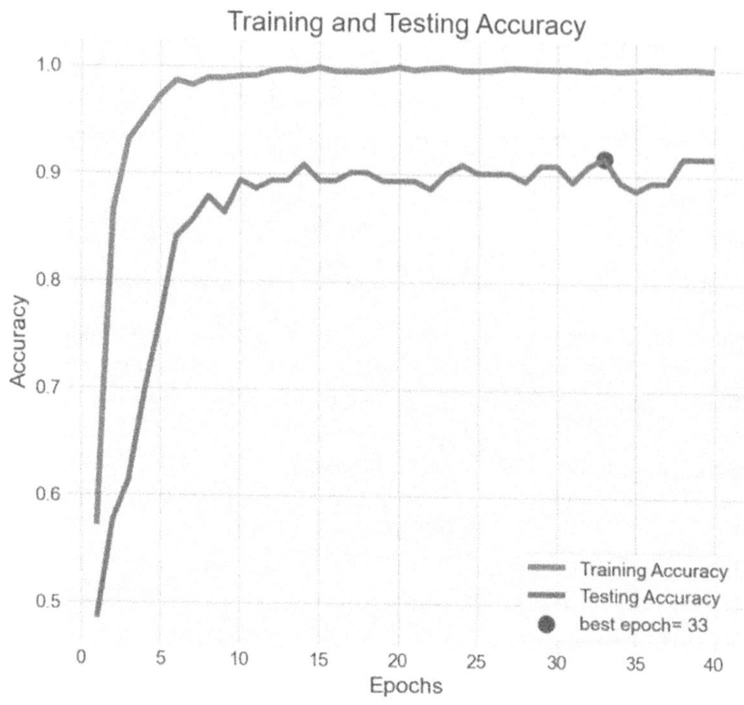

Figure 9. Accuracy graph of training and testing

generator functions, data streams were created. Fine-tuning EfficientNetB5's pre-trained model involved feeding data streams while tracking metrics like accuracy.

The model achieved a 91.66% testing accuracy, indicating proficient bone marrow cell image classification. The study also evaluated existing deep learning techniques in digital cytology, addressing drawbacks of manual cytology. Deep learning mitigates subjectivity, enhances consistency, and offers scalability, automation, and remote expertise through telepathology, transforming cytology's diagnostic potential.

Manual cytology's limitations stem from subjectivity, labor-intensiveness, and inter-observer variability, affecting accuracy and accessibility. In contrast, deep learning leverages digitization and whole slide imaging, efficiently processing vast cytological data. Convolutional neural networks (CNNs) extract features from digitized slides, improving speed and precision. By learning from extensive annotated datasets, deep learning reduces variability and enhances diagnostic consistency. Automated, objective classification minimizes reliance on human interpretation, while telepathology bridges expertise gaps in remote areas.

In summary, deep learning's integration into digital cytology enhances accuracy, scalability, and accessibility. By addressing manual cytology's challenges, deep learning paves the way for advanced disease diagnosis and screening, transforming the field's capabilities.

While Deep Learning algorithms have demonstrated better performances compared to traditional statistical methods in cytology, there is still room for improvement, as discussed in the literature review section of this work and by other researchers. The authors acknowledge the potential enhancements that can be made to their approach. One such improvement involves utilizing a larger dataset, augmented by extensive medical data. By incorporating more diverse and comprehensive data, the model's performance can be further enhanced.

Moreover, the authors used a pre-trained model that had a general-purpose design. To achieve even better results, it is suggested to explore and employ models specifically tailored for classifying bone marrow cells. These specialized models may possess a deeper understanding of the domain, resulting in improved accuracy and robustness.

Additionally, the authors recognize the potential of employing other deep learning techniques in conjunction with their proposed approach. As medical data continues to grow in size and complexity, leveraging advanced techniques can help handle and extract valuable insights from the data more effectively.

In summary, the authors acknowledge the scope for improvement in their work, including the utilization of a larger dataset with more extensive medical information, the exploration of specialized models, and the integration of other deep learning techniques to handle the evolving challenges posed by complex medical data.

References

[1] Matek, C., Krappe, S., Münzenmayer, C., Haferlach, T. and Marr, C. Highly accurate differentiation of bone marrow cell morphologies using deep neural networks on a large image data set. Blood, The Journal of the American Society of Hematology, 138(20): 1917-1927, 2021.

[2] Fu, X., Fu, M., Li, Q., Peng, X., Lu, J., Fang, F. et al. Morphogo: An automatic bone marrow cell classification system on digital images analyzed by artificial intelligence. Acta Cytologica, 64(6): 588-596, 2020.

[3] Tayebi, R.M., Mu, Y., Dehkharghanian, T., Ross, C., Sur, M., Foley, R. et al. Automated bone marrow cytology using deep learning to generate a histogram of cell types. Communications Medicine, 2(1): 45, 2022.

[4] Ananthakrishnan, B., Shaik, A., Akhouri, S., Garg, P., Gadag, V. and Kavitha, M.S. Automated bone marrow cell classification for haematological disease diagnosis using siamese neural network. Diagnostics, 13(1): 112, 2022.

[5] Yu, Z., Li, J., Wen, X., Han, Y., Jiang, P., Zhu, M. et al. AMLnet, A deep-learning pipeline for the differential diagnosis of acute myeloid leukemia from bone marrow smears. Journal of Hematology & Oncology, 16(1): 27, 2023.

[6] Wang, M., Dong, C., Gao, Y., Li, J., Han, M.. and Wang, L. A deep learning model for the automatic recognition of aplastic anemia, myelodysplastic syndromes, and

acute myeloid leukemia based on bone marrow smear. Frontiers in Oncology, 12, 2022.

[7] Choi, J.W., Ku, Y., Yoo, B.W., Kim, J.A., Lee, D.S., Chai, Y.J. et al. White blood cell differential count of maturation stages in bone marrow smear using dual-stage convolutional neural networks. PloS One, 12(12): e0189259, 2017.

[8] Song, T.H., Sanchez, V., Daly, H.E. and Rajpoot, N.M. Simultaneous cell detection and classification in bone marrow histology images. IEEE Journal of Biomedical and Health Informatics, 23(4): 1469-1476, 2018.

[9] Chandradevan, R., Aljudi, A.A., Drumheller, B.R., Kunananthaseelan, N., Amgad, M., et al. Machine-based detection and classification for bone marrow aspirate differential counts: Initial development focusing on nonneoplastic cells. Laboratory Investigation, 100(1): 98-109, 2020.

[10] Kimura, K., Tabe, Y., Ai, T., Takehara, I., Fukuda, H., Takahashi, H. et al. A novel automated image analysis system using deep convolutional neural networks can assist to differentiate MDS and AA. Scientific Reports, 9(1): 1-9, 2019.

[11] Wu, Y.Y., Huang, T.C., Ye, R.H., Fang, W.H., Lai, S.W. Chang, P.Y. et al. A hematologist-level deep learning algorithm (BMSNet) for assessing the morphologies of single nuclear balls in bone marrow smears: Algorithm development. JMIR Medical Informatics, 8(4): e15963, 2020.

[12] Liu, J., Yuan, R., Li, Y., Zhou, L., Zhang, Z. et al. A deep learning method and device for bone marrow imaging cell detection. Annals of Translational Medicine, 10(4): 2022.

[13] Stumpf, P.S., Du, X., Imanishi, H., Kunisaki, Y., Semba, Y., Noble, T. et al. Transfer learning efficiently maps bone marrow cell types from mouse to human using single-cell RNA sequencing. Communications Biology, 3(1): 736, 2020.

[14] Roy, S.S., Pratyush, C. and Barna, C. Predicting ozone layer concentration using multivariate adaptive regression splines, random forest and classification and regression tree. *In:* Soft Computing Applications: Proceedings of the 7th International Workshop Soft Computing Applications (SOFA 2016), Volume 2 7, 140-152, 2018. Springer International Publishing.

[15] Wang, C.W., Huang, S.C., Lee, Y.C., Shen, Y.J., Meng, S.I. and Gaol, J.L. Deep learning for bone marrow cell detection and classification on whole-slide images. Medical Image Analysis, 75: 102270, 2022.

[16] Bose, A., Roy, S.S., Balas, V.E. and Samui, P. Deep learning for brain computer interfaces. Handbook of Deep Learning Applications, 333-344, 2019.

[17] Roy, S.S. and Taguchi, Y.H. Identification of genes associated with altered gene expression and m6A profiles during hypoxia using tensor decomposition based unsupervised feature extraction. Scientific Reports, 11(1): 8909, 2021.

[18] Chakraborty, C., Bhattacharya, M., Sharma, A.R., Roy, S.S., Islam, M.A., Chakraborty, S. et al. Deep learning research should be encouraged for diagnosis and treatment of antibiotic resistance of microbial infections in treatment associated emergencies in hospitals. International Journal of Surgery, 105: 106857, 2022.

[19] Roy, S.S., Krishna, P.V. and Yenduri, S. Analyzing intrusion detection system: An ensemble based stacking approach. *In:* 2014 IEEE International Symposium on Signal Processing and Information Technology (ISSPIT), 000307-000309, 2014, December. IEEE.

[20] Roy, S.S., Roy, A., Samui, P., Gandomi, M. and Gandomi, A.H. Hateful Sentiment Detection in Real-Time Tweets: An LSTM-Based Comparative Approach. IEEE Transactions on Computational Social Systems. 2023.

[21] Parthvi, A., Rawal, K. and Choubey, D.K. A Comparative study using Machine Learning and Data Mining Approach for Leukemia. 2020 International Conference on Communication and Signal Processing (ICCSP), Chennai, India, pp. 0672-0677, 2020, doi: 10.1109/ICCSP48568.2020.9182142.

[22] Choubey, D.K., Raj, S., Aman, A., Deoli, R. and Hanselia, R. Detection of malaria by using a CNN model. *In:* Sisodia, D.S., Garg, L., Pachori, R.B., Tanveer, M. (eds), Machine Intelligence Techniques for Data Analysis and Signal Processing. Lecture Notes in Electrical Engineering, vol. 997. 2023. Springer, Singapore. https://doi.org/10.1007/978-981-99-0085-5_57

[23] Agarwal, D., Agarwal, R., Choubey, D.K. and Shukla, V. Design and implementation of IoT-based medicine dispensary box. *In:* Nath, V., Mandal, J.K. (eds), Microelectronics, Communication Systems, Machine Learning and Internet of Things. Lecture Notes in Electrical Engineering, vol. 887. 2023. Springer, Singapore. https://doi.org/10.1007/978-981-19-1906-0_31

[24] Choubey, D.K., Kumar, A., Srivastava, K. and Pahari, S. Notification and image analysis in cloud. *In:* 2020 International Conference on Emerging Trends in Information Technology and Engineering (ic-ETITE), pp. 1-5, 2020, February. IEEE.

[25] Choubey, D.K., Gupta, A., Suvvari, S. and Pathak, N. IoT driven precision cultivation for diverse Indian climate conditions. Soft Computing: Theories and Applications, 275-282, 2022. Springer, Singapore.

[26] Jangir, S.K., Joshi, N., Kumar, M., Choubey, D.K., Singh, S. and Verma, M. Functional link convolutional neural network for the classification of diabetes mellitus. International Journal for Numerical Methods in Biomedical Engineering, 37(8): e3496, 2021.

[27] Choubey, D.K., Paul, S. and Dhandhania, V.K. GA_NN: An intelligent classification system for diabetes. Soft Computing for Problem Solving: SocProS 2017, 2: 11-23, 2019. Springer Singapore.

[28] Choubey, D.K., Paul, S., Bala, K., Kumar, M. and Singh, U.P. Implementation of a hybrid classification method for diabetes. *In:* Intelligent Innovations in Multimedia Data Engineering and Management, 201-240, 2019. IGI Global.

[29] Choubey, D.K. and Paul, S. GA_SVM: A classification system for diagnosis of diabetes. Handbook of Research on Soft Computing and Nature-Inspired Algorithms, 359-397, 2017. IGI Global.

Index

A

Accuracy, 184, 185, 187, 188, 189, 191-193, 200
Artificial Intelligence (AI), 144, 146, 150
AUC, 190, 192, 193, 197, 199, 200

B

Big data analytics, 1, 2
Bioconductor packages, 18, 29
Bone marrow cell, 184-187

C

Cardiovascular and deep learning, 166
Chest X-ray images, 111, 112, 124, 126
Cloud computing, 1, 2
CNN, 184, 186, 188, 189, 191, 193, 196, 198, 205
Convolution neural networks, 68, 110, 112-116, 123
COVID-19 diagnosis, 110, 113, 124
Cybersecurity, 144-146, 153-155
Cytology, 184, 191, 212

D

Data analysis, 167, 171
Deep learning, 52, 53, 61, 67, 68, 71, 187, 204, 205, 212
Disease diagnosis, 76, 77

E

ECG, 166-175
Ethical considerations, 31, 41
Extract, transform and load paradigm, 61

G

Gaussian distribution, 134
Genomic science, 18
Genomics, 131

H

Healthcare analytics, 31-34, 36, 38, 43
Healthcare, 76-78, 144-147, 149-160

I

Increasing data availability, 131
Industry 4.0, 1, 2, 10
Informatics, 1, 2, 10
Internet of Medical Things (IoMT), 146
Internet of Things (IoT) technology, 126
Internet of Things (IoT), 1-5, 10, 31, 52, 76, 77, 144, 145, 147, 157, 167

M

Machine learning (ML), 1-4, 10, 31, 76-78, 81

P

Pandemic management, 110, 126
Particle swarm optimization, 59
Patient-centred care, 76, 87, 93
Patient-centric approaches, 31
Personalized treatment, 76, 77, 84

Predictive healthcare, 32

R

Radio frequency identification, 56
Remote Patient Monitoring (RPM), 76, 77, 86

S

Security considerations, 31

T

Tanmer-Whitehouse method, 71
TDbasedUFE, 18-21
TDbasedUFEadv, 18, 20, 24
Tensor decomposition, 18, 131, 136, 137
Time division multiple access, 56

U

Unsupervised feature extraction, 18

W

Wireless sensor network, 53

For Product Safety Concerns and Information please contact our EU representative GPSR@taylorandfrancis.com
Taylor & Francis Verlag GmbH, Kaufingerstraße 24, 80331 München, Germany

www.ingramcontent.com/pod-product-compliance
Lightning Source LLC
LaVergne TN
LVHW010559110826
845149LV00003B/705

* 9 7 8 1 0 3 2 5 4 4 5 7 1 *